Chapter 15 ? 66

Chapter 16 68

Chapter 17 Other goodies and factoids 74

Chapter 18 How to Overcome Food Addiction 76

Chapter 19 Techniques to Eliminate Food Addictions 106

Chapter 20 A Week of Meals to Break Your Junk Food Addiction 121

Chapter 21 Mind Tricks to Beat Your Food Addiction and Stop Emotional Eating 126

Chapter 22 Mind Tricks 128

Food Addiction

How to Stick With Your Diet Without Binging Ever Again

Doris J Barnes

Table of Contents

Chapter 1 What is addiction?..1

Chapter 2 What is food addiction?..............................2

Chapter 3 Understanding about Food Addiction ..7

Chapter 4 Food Addiction Treatment, Signs and Causes 22

Chapter 5 Defining Food Addiction 25

Chapter 6 When Eating Becomes Food Addiction 28

Chapter 7 Signs and Symptoms................................. 32

Chapter 8 Causes of Food Addiction 41

Chapter 9 Treatment for Food Addiction.............. 45

Chapter 10 How Does Food Addiction Occur In The Brain? 46

Chapter 11 What Are The Effects of Food Addiction?.. 49

Chapter 12 Treating Food Addiction 51

Chapter 13 The Basis of Food Addiction Treatment and Recovery 52

Chapter 14 Tips for a Successful Recovery from Food Addiction 53

Chapter 1
What is addiction?

Addiction is an overpowering craving to repeatedly participate in an action that gives impermanent alleviation to the detriment of repulsive consequences. It's something you feel constrained to do, despite the fact that it hurts you.

To consider an addiction, there must also be withdrawal feelings of discomfort, misery, and intense cravings when our addictive substance or behavior is taken away or stopped.

Chapter 2
What is food addiction?

Food is basic to human survival and is a critical aspect of our wellbeing, in addition to a method for pleasure and enjoyment. Food not just gives required sustenance, it also includes a gratification factor through different tastes, smells, surfaces, and so on. However, for some individuals, food can become as addictive as drugs are to a substance abuser. For men and women suffering with a food addiction, profoundly palatable foods (which are often rich in fat, sugar, as well as salt) trigger concoction reactions in the brain that induce feelings of pleasure and satisfaction. This reaction has been explained as similar to an addicts response to their substance of decision, as it activates a similar brain remunerate focus.

Food addicts become subordinate upon the "great" feelings that are obtained from consuming certain foods, which often perpetuates a continued need to eat, notwithstanding when not eager. These behaviors generate an endless loop of food addiction. As the food someone who is addicted continues to glut upon foods that induce pleasurable feelings, they often overindulge and eat beyond what is required for satiety and typical nutrition. This can prompt to a few physical, emotional, and social consequences, for example, stomach related problems, coronary illness, obesity, low–self esteem, depression, and isolation. A food someone who is addicted will often re-take part in these damaging behaviors, even amidst undesired consequences, because of the requirement for induced feelings of pleasure. Because of the fierce cycle of food addiction and the detrimental consequences associated with this behavior, it is urgent that professional food addiction help is looked for. If you or a friend or family member has been struggling with an addiction to food, consider the conceivable outcomes of a life free of this weight. You can find peace from a food addiction by seeking the appropriate care and help you require.

Food addiction is a disorder portrayed by preoccupation with food, the accessibility of food and the anticipation of pleasure from the ingestion of food. Food addiction involves the monotonous consumption of food against the individual's better judgment resulting in loss of control and preoccupation or the restriction of food and preoccupation with body weight and picture. Anorexia Nervosa is described by intense dread of gaining weight. Bulimia Nervosa is described as binge eating and compensatory behavior to forestall weight gain. Urgent Overeaters utilize food inappropriately and in the long run become dependent on it and lose control over the measure of food they eat.

Food addiction is, basically, being dependent on garbage food in an indistinguishable path from drug addicts are dependent on drugs.

It involves similar areas in the brain, similar neurotransmitters and a significant number of the symptoms are indistinguishable.

Food addiction is a relatively new (and controversial) term and there are no great statistics accessible on how common it is.

This is fundamentally the same as a few other eating disorders, including binge eating disorder, bulimia, enthusiastic overeating and having an "unhealthy" relationship with food.

Subsequently, food addiction involves a consistent compulsion to eat or potentially consume specific foods, despite the fact that those foods hurt us whether that's because the foods are unhealthy (e.g. high in sugar), or because they make us wiped out, or make us become obese.

An occasional huge feast: not addiction. Frequently eating so much, thus quickly, that you wind up bloated and nauseated but feel not able to stop? Potential addiction.

After having a couple of treats (or any potentially addictive food), a non-someone who is addicted will feel indifferent about eating more. The experience of a fiend is entirely different. Addicts become totally single-minded in the quest for their "hit". Eating a couple of treats (or any potentially addictive food) sets off an irregular reaction – and they need increasingly until they're physically not able to swallow.

If you aren't a someone who is addicted, it isn't so much that you are a master of self–control, you simply don't have an insatiable hunger for additional.

A food junkie can be:

> •an overweight lady who is continually trying another diet

> •a man who eats beyond totality at dinner after snacking on garbage food throughout the day to help manage job push

> •a thin lady who never eats enough and is ravenous all the time because she's apprehensive about getting fat (in this case, her "hit" is not eating)

> •a lonely person with nothing to do on a Friday night except watch TV and eat a few packs of chips

> •a person who snacks throughout the day to ease the fatigue of an un–stimulating life

> •a perfectionist who is never entirely satisfied with their body

•a person suffering from a nutrition related disease (e.g., coronary illness, diabetes, and so forth.) who gets disturbingly safe when given treatment approaches

Some food addicts eat too much; some don't consume enough. For a food someone who is addicted, food gives the fun, entertainment, control, reassurance, or love that's missing in their life. Food may also numb difficult emotions like dread and pity. Some individuals even have addiction to restriction.

Chapter 3
Understanding about Food Addiction

The possibility that a person can be dependent on food has as of late gained increasing support. That originates from brain imaging and other investigations of the effects of impulsive overeating on pleasure centers in the brain.

Experiments in creatures and people show that, for some individuals, a similar reward and pleasure centers of the brain that are activated by addictive drugs like cocaine and heroin are also activated by food, particularly exceptionally palatable foods. Very palatable foods will be foods rich in:

- •Sugar

- •Fat

- •Salt

Like addictive drugs, profoundly palatable foods trigger feel–great brain chemicals, for example, dopamine. Once individuals experience pleasure associated with increased dopamine transmission in the brain's reward pathway from eating certain foods, they rapidly feel the need to eat again.

The reward signals from exceedingly palatable foods may override other signs of completion and satisfaction. Subsequently, individuals continue eating, notwithstanding when they're not eager. Enthusiastic overeating is a sort of behavioral addiction meaning that someone can become preoccupied with a behavior, (for example, eating, or gambling, or shopping) that triggers intense pleasure. Individuals with food addictions lose control over their eating behavior and find themselves spending extreme measures of time involved with food and overeating, or anticipating the emotional effects of enthusiastic overeating.

Individuals who show signs of food addiction may also build up a kind of tolerance to food. They eat to an ever increasing extent, only to find that food satisfies them less and less.

Researchers believe that food addiction may assume an essential part in obesity. But typical weight individuals may also battle with food addiction. Their bodies may just be hereditarily customized to better handle the additional calories they take in. Then again they may increase their physical action to compensate for overeating.

Individuals who are dependent on food will continue to eat despite negative consequences, for example, weight gain or harmed relationships. Furthermore, like individuals who are dependent on drugs or gambling, individuals who are dependent on food will experience difficulty stopping their behavior, regardless of the possibility that they need to or have attempted ordinarily to decrease.

Help for Food Addiction

Science is as yet working to understand and find treatments for food addiction.

Some contend that recovery from food addiction might be more complicated than recovery from other kinds of addictions. Heavy drinkers, for example, can ultimately abstain from drinking liquor. But individuals who are dependent on food still need to eat.

A nutritionist, clinician, or doctor who is educated about food addiction might be ready to help you break the cycle of urgent overeating.

There are also a growing number of projects that help individuals who are dependent on food. Some, like Food Addicts in Recovery Anonymous, are based on the 12–stage program that has helped many individuals dependent on liquor, drugs, or gambling.

Others, like Food Addicts Anonymous, utilize the principles of the 12–stage program along with strict diets that encourage individuals to abstain from problem ingredients, like sugar, refined flour, and wheat.

Food Addiction is a Serious Problem

Although the expression "addiction" is often thrown around lightly, having genuine addiction is not kidding business.

I'm a recovering alcoholic, smoker and drug fanatic with a history of numerous recoveries, imprison more often than I can check and a few treks to the crisis room due to overdose.

After I had been sober for quite a long while, I began to build up an addiction to unhealthy foods.

Out and out addiction. Nothing all the more, nothing less.

The reason I'm telling you this is to demonstrate that I know how addiction works.

I'm here to reveal to you that food addiction is the same as addiction to drugs… precisely the same.

The symptoms and thought procedures are totally indistinguishable. It's only a different substance and the social consequences aren't as extreme.

Food addiction can bring about physical damage. It can lead genuine diseases like obesity, sort 2 diabetes, coronary illness, cancer, Alzheimer's, joint inflammation and depression, to give some examples.

But you have considerably greater reasons to stop than some new disease in your inaccessible future. Food addiction is also ruining your life… today.

It breaks your self–esteem, makes you unhappy with your body and can make your life a living damnation (like it accomplished for me).

The earnestness of being a food someone who is addicted can not be overstated. This is a problem that ruins lives and murders individuals. Truly.

The Law of Addiction – Why You May Never be Able to Eat "Typically" Again

The most critical lesson I have ever learned is known as the law of addiction:

"Administration of a drug to a fiend will bring about reestablishment of concoction reliance upon the addictive substance."

A former smoker who has a puff of a cigarette will become dependent again… instantly.

A drunkard who has a taste of beer will backslide, with all the ghastly consequences that follow.

There is no chance to get of getting around it. This is just how addiction works.

I am personally convinced that food addiction is the same. One nibble of cake, one taste of coke, one "cheat" – that's all it takes.

Obviously, we as a whole need to eat something. Otherwise amazing starvation. But nobody needs to eat sugar, refined wheat flour or any of the advanced garbage foods that individuals have a tendency to lose control over.

Most food addicts will never be ready to eat garbage food like "customary" individuals again. That's the frosty, hard truth.

But if they figure out how to stay away from the "trigger foods," then they ought to be ready to eat healthy and get in shape without problems.

In all actuality... finish abstinence is the only thing that dependably works against addiction. The sooner you acknowledge that, the sooner you will recover.

Although the "everything in moderation" message may work for some individuals, this advice is a total disaster for food addicts.

With regards to addiction, moderation falls flat. Without fail.

This is the basic (but difficult) solutio to addiction. Avoiding the addictive substance at all circumstances.

How to Know if This is Worth The SacrificeTotally avoiding garbage foods may appear to be incomprehensible.

These foods are everywhere and are a noteworthy piece of our way of life.

But believe me... once you've settled on the decision to never eat them again, avoiding them really becomes easier.

When you've settled on a firm decision to stay away from them totally, then there's no requirement for you to justify anything in your mind and the cravings may not show up.

Many individuals who have done this (including myself) don't get cravings any longer, not after they've settled on a profound decision to just maintain a strategic distance from this stuff... permanently.

But if you're still in doubt and are uncertain if this is justified regardless of the sacrifice, then record a rundown of advantages and disadvantages.

> •Pros may include: I'll get thinner, I'll live longer, I'll have more vitality and feel better each day, and so on.

> •Cons may include: I won't be ready to eat frozen yogurt with my family, no treats on Christmas, I may need to explain my food decisions... (Most of these social dilemmas can be solved easily).

Compose everything down, regardless of how particular or vain. At that point put your two records next to each other and ask yourself: Is it justified, despite all the trouble?

If the appropriate response is a resounding "yes" – then you can rest assured that you are doing the right thing.

Get ready Yourself and Set a Date

There are a couple of things you can do to plan yourself and make the transition as easy as conceivable: •Trigger Foods: Write down a rundown of the foods you have a tendency to desire and additionally binge on. These are the "trigger foods" you have to keep away from totally.

> •Fast Food Places: Write down a rundown of fast food places that serve healthy foods. This is vital and can keep a backslide when you find yourself hungry and not in the state of mind to cook.

> •What to Eat: Think about what foods you're going to eat. Ideally healthy foods that you like and are as of now eating consistently.

> •Pros and Cons: Consider making a few duplicates of your "upsides and downsides" list. Keep a duplicate in your kitchen, glove compartment and satchel/wallet. Sometimes you will require a reminder about why you're doing this.

It's vital to NOT go on a "diet." Put weight reduction on hold for at least 1–3 months.

Overcoming food addiction is sufficiently hard as it is, by adding hunger and additional restrictions to the blend you will simply make things significantly harder and set yourself up for disappointment.

Presently... set a date, some time in the near future (maybe this end of the week or one week from now).

From this day and onward, you will never touch the addictive foods again. Not a single nibble, ever. Period.

At the point when All Else Fails... Seek Help

If you wind up relapsing and losing control over your consumption again, then you're not alone.

Backslides are the manage with regards to addiction, not the exception.

The vast majority have a history of a few fizzled attempts before they figure out how to prevail in the long run.

That's how it was for me and most recovering food addicts I know.

But if you backslide often, then there truly is no point in trying to do it on your own again. If you've bombed a hundred circumstances, then the odds of you succeeding when you attempt it for the 101th time are practically nonexistent.

Fortunately, help is not far–removed...

There are health professionals and support groups that can help you overcome this difficult problem.

You can look for professional help… for example from a therapist or psychiatrist. Attempt to find someone who has genuine encounter in dealing with food addiction.

Simply go to their sites, find a meeting (they also have online Skype meetings) and go to it.

On the other hand you can utilize google to find treatment options in your general vicinity. Search for something like "food addiction treatment [name of city]" – odds are that you will find something that suits you.

What are warning signs for anorexia nervosa?

Behaviors associated with Anorexia Nervosa include unnecessary weighing, over the top measuring of body parts, and persistently using a mirror to check body estimate. Self–esteem is needy upon body shape and weight. Weight reduction is seen as a great achievement and an example of extraordinary self–discipline. Persons with Anorexia Nervosa may create odd and ceremonial eating propensities, for example, cutting their food into tiny pieces, refusing to eat in front of others, or fixing elaborate dinners for others that they themselves don't eat.

What are the effects of anorexia nervosa?

Physical implication of Anorexia Nervosa may include disruption of the menstrual cycle, signs of starvation, thinning of hair or male pattern baldness, bloated feeling, yellowish palms/soles of feet, dry, pasty skin. Starvation experienced by persons with Anorexia Nervosa can make harm imperative organs, for example, the heart, kidneys, and brain. Additional complications may include drop in heartbeat rate and circulatory strain, sporadic heart rhythms or heart disappointment. Nutritional deprivation may also prompt to fragile bones and osteoporosis, decreased brain volume, death by suicide or complications of the malnutrition.

What are warning signs of bulimia nervosa?

Individuals with Bulimia Nervosa become ashamed of their eating behavior and attempt to conceal symptoms through fast consumption of food. They will eat until painfully full and stop if intruded upon. 80–90% of bulimics will induce vomiting. Other behaviors include abuse of laxative, diuretics, fasting, over the top work out, and hoarding of food. A discouraged state of mind and loss of sexual interest are common among bulimics, as is continuous complaints of sore throats and abdominal pains.

What are the effects of bulimia nervosa?

Physical implication of Bulimia Nervosa may include loss of dental veneer, increase of holes, swollen spit organs, calluses, scars on hands (from self induced vomiting), sporadic menstrual cycle, reliance on laxatives for defecations, liquid and electrolyte unsettling influence. Individuals with Bulimia Nervosa, despite the fact that of ordinary weight, can extremely harm their bodies by incessant binging and purging. Malnutrition, like Anorexia Nervosa, may prompt to cardiac complications, heart disappointment, stomach rupture, or sudden death.

What are the warning signs of urgent overeating?

Overeaters demonstrate uncontrollable binge eating without extraordinary weight control and see that behavior as typical. Overeaters give moderate to extreme obesity, with a normal binge eater being 60% overweight. Binge–eating scenes consist of carbohydrates and garbage food with most binges done in booked mystery.

Food Addiction Effects

If you or your cherished one had been struggling with a food addiction, you may understand the implications this may have on the different aspects of your life. If a food addiction is left disregarded or untreated, it can quickly begin consuming your life, creating damaging and chronic symptoms. Understanding how food addiction may affect the different aspects of your life may urge you to get the help you require and merit. The following are some of the effects of food addiction:

Physical Effects – A food addiction can bring about many negative physical consequences on the body as an overabundance of food is consumed. These are some physical effects that might be experienced:

- Heart disease
- Diabetes
- Digestive Problems
- Malnutrition
- Obesity
- Chronic fatigue
- Chronic pain
- Sleep disorders
- Reduced sex drive
- Headaches
- Lethargy
- Arthritis
- Stroke
- Kidney/Liver Disease
- Osteoporosis

Mental Effects – Food addiction can be debilitating to mental health, particularly if there is absence of support or inadequate offer assistance. Some of the mental effects that might be experienced include:

- Low self–esteem

- Depression

- Panic attacks

- Increased feelings of anxiety

- Feeling tragic, sad, or in despondency

- Increased crabbiness, particularly if access to fancied food is limited

- Emotional detachment or deadness

- Suicidal ideation

Finally, food addiction can affect your social life and relationships. Social effects of food addiction include:

- Decrease performance at work or school

- Isolation from friends and family

- Division within families

- Lack of enjoyment in side interests or exercises once appreciated

- Avoidance of social occasions or functions

•Risk of jeopardizing finances or career

Chapter 4
Food Addiction Treatment, Signs and Causes

Food is not just a need of life it's also a wellspring of pleasure and a method for social engagement.

We utilize food to comfort ourselves, to sustain our friends and family, and to celebrate our occasions and extraordinary occasions. But for some individuals, the need to consume food becomes enthusiastic and uncontrollable. In these individuals, food transforms into a wellspring of addiction. Although they may attempt to control their addictive behavior through dieting or self–regulation, they tend to swing back to overeating in response to stress, outrage, or emotional pain.

Unlike liquor or illegal drugs, food is important for physical survival. However like drugs and liquor, food triggers brain chemicals that create feelings of pleasure and comfort, like dopamine, a neurotransmitter that assumes an imperative part in the brain's natural reward framework. For individuals who experience the ill effects of food addiction, consuming extensive quantities of food for the most part exceedingly palatable foods rich in fat, sugar, or starch initially offers a surge of pleasurable sensations or a release from emotional trouble. However these positive responses are soon followed by feelings of disgrace, blame, and physical discomfort. Professional treatment is often required to break the cycle of addictive overeating and restore a healthy relationship to food.

The Centers for Disease Control and Prevention has found that 35 percent of adults in the US are obese, indicating that overeating is a genuine threat to general health. Although food addiction can certainly prompt to weight gain, not everyone who experiences this disorder is obese or even overweight. An investigation of adults of varying weights distributed in Frontiers in Psychiatry uncovered the following outcomes:

- •10 percent of underweight respondents met the criteria for food addiction

- •6.3 percent of ordinary weight respondents met the criteria

- •14 percent of overweight respondents met the indicative criteria

- •Over 33% of obese respondents met the symptomatic criteria

It is interesting to note that in this review test, food addiction was more common among underweight individuals than among typical weight respondents. Rather than looking at individuals' weights or body sorts to determine whether they have a problem with food addiction, the diary focuses on that it is essential to take a gander at behaviors, for example, habitual eating, the inability to stop addictive food behaviors, and feelings of low self–worth or regret after overeating.

Chapter 5
Defining Food Addiction

"Addiction"is as a rule associated with substances that are potentially unsafe or illegal, for example, liquor, tobacco, or road drugs. However, in some cases, the brain and body can become reliant on healthy substances like food. Like liquor abuse or drug reliance, food addiction can be described by the following addictive behaviors:

•Obsessive food cravings, combined with a preoccupation with obtaining and consuming food

•The continued abuse of food (through binge eating or urgent overeating) disregarding genuine health consequences

•Repeated attempts to stop overeating, followed by backslide into addictive behaviors

•Loss of control over how much, how often, and where overeating happens

•A negative impact on work, family life, financial status, or social exercises accordingly of overeating

•The need to consume more food with a specific end goal to get a similar feeling of emotional release or comfort

•A pattern of eating alone keeping in mind the end goal to evade negative attention from others

From the get go, food addiction may appear to be relatively safe contrasted with an addiction to liquor, cocaine, methamphetamine, or heroin. However, habitual overeating can take a serious toll on physical and emotional health.

Addictive food consumption often concentrates on foods that are high in sugar, fat, or salt all of which are thick in calories and potentially destructive to the health of the heart. The health dangers of food addiction include:

•Obesity

•Diabetes

•High cholesterol

•High circulatory strain

•Heart disease

•An increased danger of stroke or heart attack

•Depression

•Social isolation

Individuals who battle with food addiction may also utilize drugs or liquor to numb feelings of depression and low self-worth. The continuous effort and inability to control urgent eating or binging can bring about feelings of sadness or misery that may even prompt to self-destructive thoughts or suicide attempts.

Chapter 6
When Eating Becomes Food Addiction

In a culture where food is so generally accessible, and where eating is often used as a wellspring of entertainment or emotional comfort, overeating is normal. However, there are certain warnings that indicate that eating has become an addictive behavior rather than a healthy wellspring of nutrition or gratification:

- •Engaging in continuous binges, or the consumption of bigger than–typical quantities of food at a fast speed

- •Consistently eating to the point of physical discomfort or pain

- •Consuming food instead of working, engaging in social exercises, or spending time with family

- •Experiencing problems at work, school, or home because of overeating

- •A consistent pattern of eating in response to depression or anxiety, or to calm feelings of outrage, bitterness, or loneliness

- •Experiencing feelings of blame, regret, or self–loathing therefore of one's inability to stop overeating

Urgent overeating, followed by feelings of blame and self–loathing, happens in a few different eating disorders.

Some of these disorders involve a pattern of binge eating followed by purging through intensive food restriction, urgent work out, or self–induced vomiting, while others don't have a purging component:

•Binge eating disorder: One of the most common forms of food addiction, binge eating disorder is set apart by repeated scenes of overeating to the point of physical discomfort. These scenes, called binges, often happen in response to emotional trouble or anxiety and result in feelings of disgrace, blame, and self–loathing. The National Eating Disorders Association estimates that 3.5 percent of American women and 2 percent of American men experience the ill effects of binge eating disorder. Binge eating disorder, also known as habitual overeating, is presently included in the Diagnostic and Statistical Manual of Mental Disorders, Fifth Edition (DSM–5), the official indicative asset for mental health professionals.

•Bulimia nervosa: Like binge eating, bulimia is described by enthusiastic overeating scenes that cause blame, disgrace, and self–loathing. But unlike binge–eating disorder, individuals with bulimia feel the need to cleanse the assortment of intemperate calories. Purging may appear as vomiting, laxative mishandle, enthusiastic work out, or prohibitive eating. Because of this purging behavior, individuals with bulimia are more averse to be overweight or obese; however, the health dangers of binging and purging are serious. Visit self–induced vomiting can bring about serious dehydration, heart problems, malnutrition, harm to the teeth and gums, and even brain harm or blindness.

•Night eating syndrome: In this form of food addiction, binges happen basically late around evening time. Individuals with night eating syndrome may consume a lot of food around evening time, while feeling next to zero yearning during the day. This phenomenon might be caused by an aggravation in typical waking–sleeping rhythms; however, there is also a component of emotional release

> involved with these eating scenes. Individuals with night eating syndrome report that the condition deteriorates when they are under anxiety.

Because consuming food is such a typical piece of regular day to day existence, it is vital to be ready to distinguish between healthy eating, overeating, and food addiction. Eating in a healthy way involves choosing generally nutritious foods and consuming close to the body needs to maintain an ordinary weight. Overeating is defined as consuming more food either as far as quantity or caloric then the individual needs to fuel everyday exercises and maintain a healthy weight.

Food addiction involves a built up pattern of enthusiastic overeating, for the most part performed in isolation from others, that hinders every day functioning. With a specific end goal to meet the criteria for binge eating disorder, as defined by the DSM–5, individuals must take part in binge eating at least once every week for three months, and these scenes must bring about considerable emotional misery.

Chapter 7
Signs and Symptoms

Researchers at Yale University's Rudd Center for Food Science and Policy have built up a questionnaire to identify individuals with food addictions.

Here's a specimen of questions that can help determine if you have a food addiction. Do these actions apply to you? Do you:

Wind up eating more than planned when you begin eating certain foods

Continue eating certain foods regardless of the possibility that you're no longer ravenous

Eat to the point of feeling sick

Stress over not eating certain sorts of foods or stress over cutting down on certain sorts of foods

At the point when certain foods aren't accessible, make a special effort to obtain them

The questionnaire also asks about the impact of your relationship with food on your personal life. Ask yourself if these situations apply to you:

You eat certain foods so often or in such expansive sums that you begin eating food instead of working, spending time with the family, or doing recreational exercises.

You maintain a strategic distance from professional or social situations where certain foods are accessible because of dread of overeating.

You have problems functioning effectively at your job or school because of food and eating.

The questionnaire asks about mental withdrawal symptoms. For example, when you cut down on certain foods (excluding caffeinated beverages), do you have symptoms, for example,

Anxiety

Agitation

Other physical symptoms

The questionnaire also tries to gage the impact of food decisions on your emotions. Do these situations apply to you?

Eating food causes problems, for example, depression, anxiety, self–loathing, or blame.

You have to eat increasingly food to lessen negative emotions or increase pleasure.

Eating a similar measure of food doesn't diminish negative emotions or increase pleasure the way it used to.

Food addiction can be conspicuous by various signs and symptoms. The following are conceivable symptoms of food addiction:

Gorging in more food than one can physically tolerate

Eating to the point of feeling sick

Going out of your approach to obtain certain foods

Continuing to eat certain foods regardless of the possibility that no longer eager

Eating in secret, isolation

Avoiding social interactions, relationships, or functions to invest energy eating certain foods.

Difficulty function in a career or job because of decreased effectiveness

Spending significant measure of money on buying certain foods for binging purposes

Decreased vitality, chronic fatigue

Difficulty concentrating

Rest disorders, for example, insomnia or oversleeping

Eagerness

Fractiousness

Migraines

Stomach related disorders

Self–destructive ideations

If you or your adored one has been experiencing any of these above symptoms subsequently of food addiction, search out professional help immediately to work through these pertinent issues.

Researchers at Yale University's Rudd Center for Food Science and Policy built up a questionnaire to identify individuals with food addictions. The Yale food addiction scale includes the following:

Wind up eating more than planned when you begin eating certain foods.

Continue eating certain foods regardless of the possibility that you're no longer eager.

Eat to the point of feeling sick.

Stress over not eating certain sorts of foods or stress over cutting down on certain sorts of foods.

At the point when certain foods aren't accessible, make a special effort to obtain them.

The behavior continues despite negative medical consequences.

The questionnaire also looks to ascertained the impact of food on an individual's personal life by asking if the following applies:

You eat certain foods so often or in such extensive sums that you begin eating food instead of working, spending time with the family, or doing recreational exercises.

You maintain a strategic distance from professional or social situations where certain foods are accessible because of dread of overeating.

You have problems functioning effectively at your job or school because of food and eating.

Are all pleasurable foods automatically addictive? Most likely not.

Hyperpalatability

Prepared foods are engineered in ways that surpass basic reward properties of traditional entire foods, making them hyperpalatable.

Consider things, for example, frozen yogurt, burgers, candy, dissolved cheeses, buttery/slick sauces, et cetera – these are the foods that stimulate the release of opioids and dopamine in the brain and have addictive potential (note: artificial sweeteners can much trigger a dopamine response).

Rat examines confirm this: Rats are unlikely to binge on ordinary rat chow. But when given the option of sweeter and fattier rat chow, rats go on a bender.

The table below shows the qualities of some "ordinary" foods and some hyperpalatable foods. See how much higher in sugar, fat, as well as sodium the hyperpalatable foods are and what number ingredients every food contains.

Other things can contribute to the addictive potential of food:

Quantity: When served more, we eat more.

Processing and vitality thickness: The right blend of fat, sweeteners, flours, caffeine and salt gives a strong reward. Plain sugar parcels or a container of olive oil aren't extremely alluring. Handled foods have combinations of ingredients not found in nature. Numerous food components, like drugs, are not addictive until extricated and concentrated by present day processing (an entire grain versus white flour in cake, an entire organic product versus sugar in treats, cocaine versus cocoa leaves, opium versus poppies, and so forth.).

Assortment: When there are different hues, sizes, shapes, tastes, and surfaces, we eat more. Individuals will eat more treat batter frozen yogurt versus plain vanilla and more trail blend versus plain crude almonds.

Supplement composition of foods: When we eat supplement poor foods, we may wind up eating more overall food with a specific end goal to address supplement issues.

Get to: The number one factor in addiction is accessibility. If the substance isn't accessible, we can't build up an addiction. At the point when the substance is promptly accessible, addiction will be more common (think: cigarettes in vending machines).

Social standards: Whe a behavior/substance is acknowledged within a group, it's unlikely that behavior will stop. Numerous people cut down on or quit smoking when jurisdictions banned smoking in restaurants and bars.

Individual preferencesThink about what foods have an "addictive" potential for you. It's critical to consider these questions because any one food isn't generally "addictive."

- What foods do you want?

- What foods do you think about you aren't physically ravenous?

- What foods would you like to eat a greater amount of, notwithstanding when you're full?

- What foods do you ordinarily deny yourself of but later, feel not able to control yourself around?

- What foods have emotional associations for you say, foods you remember from childhood, or foods that appear to have "unique forces" to improve you feel?

Answers to the aforementioned questions don't more often than not include grain, pears, asparagus and dark beans (but it's conceivable).

While entire foods in their most natural form are still potentially addictive (think sweet leafy foods nuts), the potential for genuine reliance (addiction is low contrasted with handled foods, for example, organic product candies and enhanced fatty nuts).

There is no blood test accessible to analyze food addiction. Much the same as with other additions, it is based on behavioral symptoms.

Here are 8 common symptoms that are normal of food addicts:

1.You as often as possible get cravings for certain foods, despite feeling full and having recently finished a nutritious supper.

2.When you give in and begin eating a food you were craving, you often find yourself eating considerably more than you intended to.

3.When you eat a food you were craving, you sometimes eat to the point of feeling too much "stuffed."

4.You often feel blameworthy after eating specific foods, yet find yourself eating them again soon after.

5.You sometimes rationalize your mind about why you ought to eat something that you are craving.

6.You have repeatedly attempted to stop eating or setting rules (includes cheat dinners/days) about certain foods, but been unsuccessful.

7.You often shroud your consumption of unhealthy foods from others.

8.You feel not able to control your consumption of unhealthy foods despite knowing that they are causing you physical damage (includes weight gain).

Chapter 8
Causes of Food Addiction

There are a few well known hypotheses about the causes of food addiction. Researchers have determined that in certain individuals, the body's response to certain sorts of food, particularly sweet or fatty foods, is like the response to drugs or liquor. BMB Reports suggests that the compulsion to overeat emerges in a neurochemical pathway responsible for rewarding positive behaviors. Dopamine, one of the essential neurotransmitters involved in this pathway, is released in response to binge eating scenes, resulting in a high that could be contrasted with the effects of liquor or drugs.

An individual's family background may have an influence in food addiction. Individuals who originate from families where food is used as a method for reward, comfort, self–expression, or control will probably show unhealthy behaviors around food consumption in adulthood. Children who grow up watching their parents participate in overeating or incessant dieting, with periods of restriction alternating with overeating and resulting feelings of disgrace or blame, are also at danger of becoming dependent on food.

Depression, anxiety, and substance utilize disorders are common among individuals who experience the ill effects of binge eating disorder. According to Social Work Today, numerous individuals with eating disorders have a history of manhandle or injury and a propensity to swing to drugs or liquor as well as food for comfort. Social or familial weights to meet a certain physical perfect create the potential for self-perception distortion and negative feelings about one's shape or size, which can prompt to patterns of prohibitive eating and binging.

Although dieting does not bring about food addiction, prohibitive eating can definitely be a hazard factor for developing this disorder. After a period of depriving oneself of food, the body may experience a bounce back effect, in which the individual consumes a lot of calories so as to compensate for a period of food restriction. In addition to the metabolic effects of dieting, the emotional impact of food restriction may make dieters feel that they "deserve"to binge on foods that were forbidden during the diet. Those with binge eating disorder (BED), eating disorder-not otherwise specified (ED-NOS), bulimia, a family history of substance manhandle, a personal history with substance mishandle, or early life injury are generally helpless. Often, they have identifiable binge foods, for example, sugary dessert or salty snack things. Once such individuals begin consuming these binge foods, they find it nearly difficult to stop. Truth be told, if ruined for any reason, they become to a great degree on edge untilmore can be obtained, much the same as a person dependent on liquor or drugs. Food addicts continue to binge despite negative health and relationship consequences. Often, they need desperately to stop consuming these foods, but can't do as such without offer assistance. It is not strange for them to conceal food, pulverize the confirmation, for example, wrappers, or eat in secret.

Food addiction as often as possible co-happens with a disposition disorder like depression or post-traumatic anxiety disorder. Co-occurring reliance on liquor or mishandle of such substances as stimulants, cocaine, weed, benzodiazepines, or nicotine is also common

The predominance of such co-occurring disorders is what makes the professional care at Timberline Knolls Residential Treatment Center so profitable. As our clinical group helps a lady or young lady break her addiction to food, the depression, injury, substance mishandle, or other co-occurring conditions are also tended to. At Timberline Knolls, we treat all disorders and addictions all the while, knowing this offers an occupant the best conceivable shot for sustained recovery. This approach demonstrates exceptionally beneficial on a number of levels. A lady or young lady may admit to our program because of an addiction to liquor or prescription medication. Only while in treatment, may it become clear to our clinicians that she also has a food addiction. Perhaps she had shrouded this addiction for years because of disgrace or blame. Once identified, she can get the therapy required to break the addiction.

Food addiction is likely the culmination of a few factors that interplay in the overall reason for this disorder. A man or lady may build up a food addiction accordingly of organic, mental, or social reasons. Natural causes that may influence the progression of a food addiction may include hormonal irregular characteristics, variations from the norm in different brain structures, reactions from the utilization of certain medications, or having relatives with food addiction issues. A food addiction may also be the consequence of mental factors. Factors included in this category may include emotional or sexual mishandle, being a casualty or survivor of a traumatic occasion, having an inability to healthily adapt to negative situations, chronic low–self esteem, or experiencing pain or misfortune. Mental factors, for example, these can influence an individual to utilize food as a coping instrument to ease the painful emotions that may have come about. Lastly, there are social implications that might be involved with food addiction, including factors, for example, unsettling influences in family function, weight from associates or society, social isolation, child manhandle, absence of social support, and unpleasant life occasions. Food addiction can also be associated with other co–occurring disorders, for example, eating disorders or substance mishandle. Because food addiction is a complex mental health issue that can have genuine complications if left untreated, it is exceptionally recommended that professional cause be tried to effectively mend from this disorder.

Chapter 9
Treatment for Food Addiction

There are two main categories of addiction: process addiction, in which a person urgently takes part in a behavior(s) that become unmanageable; and substance addiction, in which a person habitually consumes a substance to the point that they have lost control. Food addiction falls into this latter category.

A term, for example, heroin addiction has an abnormal state of specificity; by definition, the person is dependent on one substance: heroin. The term food addiction is somewhat expansive, yet similarly substantial. The lady or young lady with this condition is dependent, with all the corresponding difficulties and negative consequences associated with any addiction. However, this individual is normally not dependent on all foods, because only certain foods have addictive qualities. These are often alluded to as calorie–thick foods. Such foods are commonly high in sugar, fat or salt. It is this abnormal state of these substances that can affect the brain in a profoundly negative fashion and cause reliance that is not unlike what we see with drug addiction. The truth of food addiction has huge implications for the individuals who battle with habitual overeating and additionally obesity, and even some individuals with binge–cleanse anorexia and bulimia.

Chapter 10
How Does Food Addiction Occur In The Brain?

The human brain is one of the most intricate, mind boggling and amazing organs in the body. However, with regards to food, it is entirely oversimplified. The brain was designed to search out those foods that the body required to propel health and sustain life. Because the brain backpedals a huge number of years, by default, these were natural foods – foods got solely from plants and creatures.

Enter the cutting edge time of manufacturing. Our faculties are assaulted every day with alluring, exceedingly handled, hyperpalatable and convenient food. It is everywhere and typically inexpensive. The problem is, such an extensive amount the fast, shoddy and extremely accessible food is not nutritionally stable by any means it is a palatable, fabricated item. These items are called hyperpalatable foods, which mean they contain inordinate measures of sugar, fat, or salt; this food is exceptionally prepared or manipulated to attract consumers and increase item deals. Unfortunately, these hyperpalatable foods cause nothing shy of mayhem in brains of individuals who are inclined to addiction. Once the path to addiction begins, it ultimately comes about a real rewiring of the brain's reward framework and related areas. The disorder begins when the brain is over saturated with these calorie–thick foods. This triggers an upgraded release of dopamine, a neuro–transmitter that motivates individuals toward food, sex, liquor, and so on. It is dopamine that gives the incredibly positive feeling when calorie–thick foods are initially consumed. But here is where the brain's original wiring enters the equation. The human brain wasn't created to adapt to a constant onslaught of hyperpalatable foods. In certain individuals, it basically cannot tolerate that level of stimulation. To secure itself, the brain diminishes the number of accessible dopamine receptors. This implies that though a lot of dopamine surge the brain, the substance is not grabbed or gotten. This receptor reduction doesn't have any significant bearing to all foods. Rat considers demonstrate it isn't recently high quantities of food, but a lot of calorie–thick food, leading to increased dopamine release, which causes the inevitable reduction in dopamine receptors. Unfortunately, what is beneficial for the brain ultimately demonstrates problematic for the consumer. To get the anticipated uplifting feedback from the food, a greater amount of the food must be onsumed to replicate the reward. Over time, the individual eats increasingly as the reward becomes less and less. This is often alluded to as "chasing the high."

In the meantime the reward focus is being captured, the prefrontal cortex, the part of the brain responsible for control, decision making and exercising judgment, is also being affected. The decrease in dopamine receptors causes decreased movement in this essential part of the brain. This implies that as more calorie–thick food is consumed to accomplish the reward, these women and young ladies are less ready to apply control over the behavior. Moderation in consumption is no longer conceivable without offer assistance. Actually, concentrates supported by the National Institutes of Health have shown that the brain scans of food addicts show an indistinguishable changes and impairments from those of a person with cocaine addiction.

Chapter 11
What Are The Effects of Food Addiction?

An addiction to food, particularly if long in duration, brings about negative consequences to all aspects of a person's life.

Physical consequences:

The transient physical effect associated with dopamine and endogenous opiate release in the brain remunerate focus is low level euphoria, a decrease in both anxiety and emotional pain. This calming, sedation experience is often alluded to as a "food trance state." The long–term physical effects shift. If the person takes part in compensatory practice, for example, purging or restricting, the health consequences can be serious. if a food fanatic has obesity, it can be associated with the following: diabetes, hypertension, elevated cholesterol and triglycerides, osteoarthritis in the knees, hips and back; contagious infections in skin overlays that are hard to perfect, congestive heart disappointment, shortness of breath, coronary conduit disease, and ultimately death.

Mental consequences:

The mental and mental effects can demonstrate intense and torment an individual for years. These include misery, feebleness, isolation, disgrace, depression, self–loathing, blame, self–destructive thoughts, suicide attempts, or potentially self-injurious behaviors.

Relational consequences:

Food addiction impacts relationships, particularly those within the family. This is because the person with the addiction is vastly more involved with food than with individuals – it becomes their most secure, most essential and meaningful relationship. Other connections to loved ones take a secondary lounge. This often prompts to a profound feeling of isolation from others. For individuals with obesity, outsiders and even friends and family often take part in bullying and shaming words and actions because of the tremendous problem our way of life has with weight disgrace. Commonly friends and family experience outrage and frustration, since they are totally not able to understand why their sister or girl just won't stop eating, particularly when it is obviously jeopardizing her health. Spouses often misperceive their wife's behaviors, believing her actions indicate she is no longer dedicated to their marriage. Such comments as "if you cherished me, you would stop binging on all that food," are normal.

Chapter 12
Treating Food Addiction

Living with any addiction is difficult and potentially life threatening. The ramifications to a person's health, career, family, and future are tremendous and often extreme. In addition, an addiction once in a while resolves on its own. A food addiction is no exception. That's the reason early intervention and treatment is imperative. Timberline Knolls Residential Treatment Center gives the care a lady or young lady needs to find flexibility. Our treatment is designed to assist restore a healthy relationship with food and allow her to come back to a life of recovery.

Chapter 13
The Basis of Food Addiction Treatment and Recovery

The individuals who have gone through professional food addiction treatment are instructed, obviously, not to abstain from food totally (that would be savage) but instead to abstain from the most addictive sorts of food.

The most addictive sorts of food are prepared foos high in sugar, fat and salt, as well as straightforward carbohydrates and sugars (white flour, refined sugar, and so forth.) It is often recommended that those in recovery from food addiction abstain from these foods, but that is a great deal more difficult than it sounds. Have a go at going to any coffee shop to get a coffee without seeing heaps of pastries, sandwiches or baked merchandise. Take a stab at doing your standard shopping for food without having to pass the bakery or garbage food passageway. For these reasons, food addiction recovery can posture many difficulties. That is the reason we have assembled a rundown of supportive tips to prop you up in food addiction recovery.

Chapter 14
Tips for a Successful Recovery from Food Addiction

To help guarantee your accomplishment in recovery, we recommend the following:

1. Attend meetings.

Attending normal meetings is basic to addiction recovery. The initial 90 days of recovery are often said to be the most difficult and during this time it might be beneficial to attend a meeting every single day if conceivable, to ensure you remain on track. Over the long haul, meetings can become less successive, but attending a meeting at least once every week is recommended throughout your whole time in recovery. Look at Food Addicts Anonymous or other comparable groups in your general vicinity. Online meetings can also be beneficial if conditions keep you from physically attending meetings.

2. Have a sponsor.

Sponsors are one of the most supportive tools you can have in an addiction recovery. Someone who has been through what you are going through and has proven to be the best can help guide you through the darkest points and help you see that achievement is conceivable, and that things will show signs of improvement. You can find a sponsor at your neighborhood meetings or by contacting your addiction treatment focus.

3. Be readied.

Be set up by continually having healthy and nutritious food in the house that is in agreement with your feast plan. Cook measured suppers early and keep them in the cooler for those bustling days that may make them long for picking up fast food to save yourself some time. If you know you have a bustling day in front of you and that you might not have room schedule–wise to take a seat at home to a healthy feast, pack something and bring it with you. Also, don't skip dinners, regardless of how bustling you are. When you are exceptionally ravenous, the scent and sight of off–point of confinement foods will be additionally tempting.

4. Keep a food diary.

A food journal or food diary is a key tool for those in food addiction recovery. It can be kept together with your dinner plan or separate, but your food diary ought to be a place to record what you ate as well as the feelings you had throughout the day. Foods that might be 'on plan' may have triggers for you that you didn't know about. One food someone who is addicted in recovery told LA Weekly that each time she ate eggs it would trigger recollections of the way her parents used to make them for her – an egg sandwich. After eating eggs she would dream of eating toast which was off points of confinement for her. Keeping a food diary can help you make associations, for example, this as well as help you understand what kind of foods make you feel your best throughout the day.

5. Know your triggers.

As beforehand mentioned, certain healthy foods may really have deeply ingrained triggers that you should keep mindful of. But those are by all account not the only triggers. If there is a specific bakery or fast food restaurant you used to visit on your approach to work that brings up cravings, it might be best to find an alternate course to work. Going to gatherings where food is served can also trigger cravings. In these cases it might be best to abstain from going to the gathering until the food is finished, or bring someone with you that knows about your recovery who can help keep you responsible and in control.

6. Keep dynamic.

Being dynamic, whether it is spending time at the rec center, joining a move class or just going for a walk every day naturally releases endorphins or 'happy hormones' that will help shield you from experiencing food cravings. That, as well as it will keep your body fit and healthy.

7. Have a backslide prevention plan.

Most food addiction treatment centers will help you make a personalized backslide prevention plan before your treatment is over, as it is integral to long and lasting recovery. A backslide prevention plan ought to include your own personal triggers, warning signs of backslide, (for example, fatigue, depression and loneliness) as well as a far reaching rundown of individuals you can converse with and actions that you can take to forestall backslide before it happens. Your sponsor ought to be ready to help you make one if you don't have one as of now.

8. Ask for help when you require it.

Conceivably the most imperative tip to effective recovery from food addiction is to not fear asking for help when you require it. If you are struggling and find yourself craving foods that are off breaking points and are anxious about the possibility that that you might be getting off track, converse with someone you trust! It is much easier to get back on track before an out and out backslide than it is afterwards.

If you or a friend or family member has gotten yourself stuck within the endless loop of a food addiction, you have likely experienced a thrill ride of emotions, including gloom, frustration, and sadness. Living with a food addiction might be preventing you from enjoying a life you once lived, though the likelihood for healing dependably exists. By seeking the appropriate help and care you require, you can find the assets to address your food addiction in an effective way. Thankfully, there are particular food addiction treatment centers that can help you approach this disorder in an all encompassing and extensive way. Food addiction treatment centers offer multi-claim to fame treatment that will concentrate on and address medical issues and nutritional concerns, while integrating psychotherapy. There are also a heap of support groups that you can become involved with, for example, Food Addicts Anonymous, Overeaters Anonymous, and Food Addicts in Recovery Anonymous. These groups are 12 stage based projects that effectively address food addiction on the physical, emotional, and profound aspects, offering genuinely necessary support to individuals seeking to recuperate from their addiction to food. Attempting to manage your food addiction alone can further draw you into dread or isolation. Having direction, help and support from an eating disorder focus that treats food addiction, master, or support group can give you or your cherished one with the tools and assets you have to recover and mend from a food addiction.

Treating food addiction is a multidimensional procedure that must address the individual's emotional, physical, and mental necessities.

Dangerous eating propensities can be hard to break, particularly if these scenes are an aftereffect of underlying mental health issues. The co-event of liquor or drug manhandle requires a component of substance mishandle treatment as well as specific attention to the eating disorder itself.

The objectives of food addiction treatment include helping the customer replace dysfunctional eating patterns with healthy ones, addressing co–occurring depression or anxiety, and helping the customer build up a stronger, more positive self–picture.

Some of the best therapeutic modalities for treating food addiction are recorded below:

•Cognitive Behavioral Therapy (CBT): CBT is a learning–based therapy that can help customers identify and change the thought patterns that prompt to overeating. In the meantime, CBT helps customers grow new coping strategies to manage the stressors and triggers that prompt to binging. CBT can be used individually, in one–on–one therapy, or in group therapy sessions with other customers who are struggling with similar issues.

•Medication: Medications used to treat depression or anxiety have been used to help control the desire to overeat. Specifically, drugs in the SSRI (particular serotonin reuptake inhibitors) category have shown positive outcomes with binge eating disorder, bulimia, and eating disorders. Prominent SSRIs include citalopram (Celexa), fluoxetine (Prozac), escitalopram (Lexapro), sertraline (Zoloft), and paroxetine

(Paxil). As an additional benefit, SSRIs can mitigate symptoms of co-occurring depression or anxiety in individuals with food addiction.

•Solution-focused therapy: This commonsense way to deal with therapy draws in customers in developing and implementing solutions to specific issues in their lives. For instance, a customer who overeats in response to work-related weight can figure out how to delegate all the more effectively or improve time management with a specific end goal to diminish the level of weight on the job.

•Trauma therapies: Overeating can be a method for figuratively "swallowing"or "stuffing down"unresolved traumas or emotional pain. Specific modalities that objective natural injury, for example, Seeking Safety or Eye Movement Desensitization Reprocessing (EMDR) can be used to help customers overcome suppressed pain so that they no longer need to overeat for comfort.

•Nutritional counseling and dietary planning: People with food addiction may need to relearn healthy eating propensities. They may also have nutritional insufficiencies thus of their eating patterns. By working with a nutritionist or enlisted dietitian, these customers can build up a healthier way to deal with making food decisions and planning suppers.

•Food addiction treatment can occur on an inpatient basis, through a private office, or in an outpatient setting at a clinic, healing facility, or recovery focus. Inpatient treatment is often recommended for individuals who have genuine co-occurring medical issues, or who have been determined to have other mental health issues or substance utilize disorders. Outpatient treatment, including intensive outpatient projects and incomplete hospitalization programs (PHPs) are appropriate for customers who have a strong support framework in place, who are motivated to seek after treatment, or who have responsibilities or obligations that keep them from staying at a treatment office fulltime.

Binge eating disorder and other forms of food addiction are becoming increasingly common in the United States. In the meantime, the health problems caused by obesity have achieved pestilence proportions. Although food addiction may not appear as genuine as drug or liquor mishandle, this disorder can bring about tremendous emotional trouble, as well as harm to the individual's physical and mental wellbeing. With compassionate, far reaching treatment, customers can figure out how to change their impulsive eating propensities and create more joyful, healthier lives.

Food dependence

But here's the problem with determining food addiction: Unlike, say, heroin or gambling, we require food to live. Without an innate longing for food, we can wave bye–bye to evolution.

At what point does "huge craving" end and "food addiction" begin? What's more, can you technically become "dependent" to something you require?

Researchers, while separated on the correct definition of "food addiction" or whether it genuinely exists, by the by concur that addiction is a pattern of behavior described by things like:

- near–constant scans for a "hit"

- an intense compulsion and additionally crave for the substance or behavior

•strong, widely inclusive concentrate on getting that "hit"

•withdrawal symptoms when the "hit" is taken away

•needing more, or more intense "hits" as tolerance creates over time

By this definition, nearly anything including food, water, or sex (i.e. things that are a piece of basic science) can be an addiction.

So how about we call it "food reliance".

Over time, food (substance) reliance often becomes less about the high and more about preventing the negative feelings that originate from abstinence. The capacity to get pleasure from the food becomes more difficult, because little measures of a similar food aren't as rewarding.

The Diagnostic and Statistical Manual of Mental Disorders (DSM–IV) defines "substance reliance" as at least 3 of the following 7 symptoms occurring within 1 year. We'll take a gander at how these might relate to food reliance.

Symptom 1: I utilize more over time.

Over time, tolerance increases.

Food example: When I used to purchase perishables, I would take them home, eat a snack and go ahead with my day. Presently I purchase perishables and I eat throughout the day until I have gone through portion of what I purchased.

Symptom 2: I have withdrawal symptoms.

I now take the substance to stay away from withdrawal.

Food example: I eat prepared snacks to right being drained as well as discouraged. To settle anxiety, I eat something crunchy, like chips or saltines to quiet myself. I am apprehensive if I stop using food to revise my emotions, I will have nothing else to swing to.

Symptom 3: I utilize more than I intend.

Food example: One bowl of frozen yogurt transforms into 2 bowls, then 3 bowls. I begin with one handful of chips and wind up eating the entire pack.

Symptom 4: I'm trying or have attempted to decrease.

I need to diminish my intake, and I've attempted, but haven't been fruitful.

Food example: I have attempted to chop down or stop my eating, but it's dependably on my mind and I find an approach to defeat myself, notwithstanding making an exceptional excursion to get a candy bar or chips.

Symptom 5: I invest energy pursuing, using, or recovering from utilize.

I invest a lot of energy in exercises important to obtain the substance, or recover from its effects.

Food example: I will have a rundown of errands to do on Saturday. I will go to the store and purchase basic needs and spend whatever remains of the day eating what I purchased, taking stomach settling agents, and sleeping.

Symptom 6: I miss imperative exercises because of my substance utilize.

I miss or surrender imperative social, occupational, or recreational exercises.

Food example: I get back home and eat. At that point, I'm too full to practice or meet with companions.

Symptom 7: I eat despite knowing the consequences.

I continue to mishandle the substance despite knowing it's giving me a persistent or intermittent physical or physiological problem.

Food example: I eat notwithstanding repulsive knee pain from obesity. I'm so uncomfortable after a binge that I can't set down without regurgitation into my throat. My circulatory strain is high. I'm hopeless. I am embarrassed and apprehensive about being in social situations but I overeat at any rate.

Chapter 15
What influences food addiction?

Many factors assume a part in the development of food addiction.

Fear: Addicts may fear eating a reasonable measure of food, getting fat, as well as experiencing uncomfortable emotions and craving.

Chronic overeating: Eating too a lot of profoundly handled foods can stimulate brain opiates "feel great" chemicals. General binging may create a reliance on this "natural high". We become reliant on an exceptionally handled diet to feel "ordinary" and experience withdrawal symptoms when we don't eat it.

Food restriction: What if I told you that starting tomorrow you would never have dessert again? What might you do today? Presumably eat a pack of frozen yogurt – right? Cravings and reward responses from food are greater after a period of food restriction (whether genuine or imagined) or potentially supplement depletion. This is the reason diets and outrageous restriction inevitably prompt to binges.

Stretch: Various forms of stress can trigger addiction. Binging + food restriction + stretch = a winning combination for food addiction. Addiction can lie lethargic when things are going admirably, then back its terrible head when life inconvenience strikes.

Depression: Depression ordinarily changes craving, yearning, and totality signals, as well as rest patterns (regularly, great quality rest helps us oversee inclinations rest is "self discipline fuel").

Powerless satiety components: Some individuals who battle with food addiction aren't as tuned in to their totality prompts. They "listen" hunger flags more uproariously than satiety signals.

Automaticity: Food behaviors can be strongly ingrained propensities that "wear a depression" into our sensory system. Some contend that they can't be eliminated quite recently rendered lethargic (briefly).

Chapter 16
Treating addiction

Individuals aren't responsible for having an addiction, but they are responsible for dealing with it.

To treat addiction, you should address the following factors:

Food accessibility and environment

If you feel wild with certain foods or in certain situations, you most likely are.

Our behavior depends intensely on social and environmental signals. We can change our behavior by adjusting prompts from our routine and environment.

Along these lines: Avoid individuals, places, and things that trigger addiction. Utilize social weight further bolstering your good fortune. Addicts don't like to utilize their drug with sober individuals staring at them.

The more accessible and socially adequate an addictive substance is, the easier it is to get snared. Make it hard to get.

Emotions

Food doesn't help resolve emotions. Furthermore, emotions aren't a terrible thing. They really fill a valuable need in life and can indicate that something is out of adjust.

Food can be used as a coping instrument for emotions that feel intolerable. Once a "food surge" wears off, we're left with the extremely same emotional problems... plus the additional problems addiction brings.

Numerous addictions come from uncontrolled anxiety combined with food restriction. If these two factors can be controlled, food addiction may also be controlled.

Pharmaceuticals

What about craving suppressants and drugs that eliminate the high from addictive foods? These purported solutions open up new problems (e.g., undereating, malnutrition, and so forth).

Consistence to pharmaceuticals like naltrexone (blocks the high someone gets from a drug) and antabuse (makes someone wiped out if they drink liquor) have a tendency to be poor. Why? Because individuals need the high again. Regardless of the possibility that a hunger suppressant drug is produced, the food addiction will at present remain. This has little to do with the addictive food itself and more to do with a deficiency elsewhere in life – fatigue, loneliness, outrage, absence of stimulation, absence of reason, and so on.

Cravings kick the bucket as a symptom of changing our life and personality medication is, at best, only a halfway and transitory solution.

However, pharmaceuticals that might be valuable in addiction recovery include those that treat underlying conditions leading to emotional trouble (pain, depression, and so on.).

Abstinence

While we can't choose to be dependent, we can choose to abstain keeping in mind the end goal to sustain recovery. Some claim that as a junkie, it's easier to surrender the addictive substance altogether than to negotiate with it.

In this case, flexibility comes when we surrender effort to control the substance and become abstinent. Recovery from addiction implies having the restoration of decision.

However, abstinence implies that addicts must be willing to face discomfort. Fortunately, the longer a fiend remains abstinent, the more organic inclinations for the substance blur. Withdrawal is most noticeably awful in the beginning.

If urges return, they're often the aftereffect of conditioned reflexes as well as the craving to escape emotional pain. Managing stress and knowing "triggers" is therefore an essential piece of recovery.

Meaning

Recovery from addiction needs meaning and reason. Without meaning, there is no reason to remain abstinent.

Outside meanings (e.g., how the body looks, a spouse, a companion) can be fleeting. We cherish them one day, hate them the following.

If we rely on outside meanings for sustained change, there's a decent shot we'll be dissatisfied. Dissatisfaction fills resentment, and soon enough we remember that overeating is a brisk approach to forget about the whole wreckage.

Meaning is one of the reasons why the possibility of a "higher power" in numerous addiction recovery projects is appealing. A higher power isn't fleeting, it's everlasting. However, what's most vital is that the meaning and reason for existing is internal it originates from the inside and mirrors the person's deeper qualities and life needs.

Getting a handle on food addiction often requires a brief hiatus from mirror and scale obsession. Instead, we should organize what's going on inside.

Dieting

Reason is no match for addiction. Addiction is for the most part an emotional–organic phenomenon.

Along these lines, addicts have a tendency to be not able depend on self–control alone which doesn't mean they are "frail". (Truth be told, given how hard most food addicts attempt to change regardless of the possibility that unsuccessfully apparently their will is exceptionally strong.)

The battle with food addiction often prompts to dieting, over–exercising, purging, drugs, binging, and weight gain/misfortune. These are efforts to control the addiction, but these efforts are often implausible, become indulgent, and in the long run come up short (and this disappointment can prompt to more addictive behaviors). Truth be told, restriction and obsession with "fixing the problem" itself can create more bounce back.

Basic changes

"Determination" helps, but it's feeble contrasted with auxiliary and foundational changes. This includes things like:

> •changing one's physical environment
>
> •building a social support framework (including getting far from individuals who empower the addiction)
>
> •making it tougher to get at the addictive substances
>
> •decreasing life stretch, as well as working on stress management
>
> •learning to tolerate discomfort, and getting support in doing so

•changing one's routine and timetable to support positive behaviors, and diminish the odds for negative behaviors (which can include things like getting more rest, seeking out more secure situations during "trigger circumstances", scheduling exercises that conflict with the addictive behavior, and so on.)

Chapter 17
Other goodies and factoids

Food addiction factoids

Compensate edge or the measure of substance expected to get a "high" increases over time. Addicts require to an ever increasing extent. In the long run, many don't get a "high" or any pleasure by any stretch of the imagination the addiction centers around managing withdrawal.

The prior we begin eating hyperpalatable foods, the more probable we are to get snared on them. This implies that great childhood nutrition is vital and handled foods focused at children are a noteworthy potential health problem.

In related factoids, the longer we're presented to innately attractive foods, the more difficult they are to stand up to. Self–control is a restricted asset. In this way, if you battle with being near certain foods, make tracks in an opposite direction from them fast. Get them out of your house, and move yourself far from them. Don't torture or entice yourself with physical vicinity.

The individuals who want to binge on sweet foods tend to binge more regularly than people who want to binge on fatty or salty foods.

Addicts often have higher levels of dopamine circulating in their brains than non–addicts. It's uncertain whether that's a cause or consequence of eating.

Binge eating (independent of body weight), rather than weight, is all the more nearly associated with addictive eating patterns. In other words, behavior predicts addiction better than body size, weight, or fatness.

Some data indicate that contrasted with women, men will probably overeat once they begin, and will probably eat more than their body needs.

Philosophical musingsIn the U.S., numerous self-dangerous compulsions are considered typical. This implies it's harder to identify problem behaviors as addictions or conditions. Indeed, if someone were to design a general public perfect for food addiction – North America would likely be it.

If we quit eating a certain food – would we say we are dependent on abstaining?

Buddhist teachings have long stated that attachment is the base of all suffering. Could this along with mindfulness training and learning to "be available" with discomfort be the way to unlocking addiction?

Chapter 18
How to Overcome Food Addiction

It's a very common situation: You get up in the morning swearing today's the day when you'll eat clean, sustain yourself with a healthy breakfast at home, and pass up the glistening bakery treats that entice you consistently.

You make it to work without incident and after that anxiety hits any kind of worry, from another project deadline to a burning comment from your manager. After a short time, you find yourself with pastries in hand, wolfing down sugary analgesics and wanting more. When you finally fly out of your food stupor, and the truth of what you've done begins to settle in, the ensuing feelings of disgrace and blame stoke your anxiety levels progressively and you're now plotting your next food settle.

You wonder: Why do I continue caving to these cravings? Where's my discipline and self control?

This is your brain dependent on food.

That's right. Dependent. You may let yourself know, "I'm not dependent on food; I simply adore a decent sweet every so often."

Indeed, I'm here to disclose to you that food addiction is genuine; it affects a larger number of individuals than you know, and makers really design food items with the goal that they are as addicting as conceivable. Yes, that perfect combination of salty, sweet, and appetizing was created to ensure you continue reaching for additional.

Here are six approaches to beat food addiction:

1) Take the test. Initially, you have to find out if your relationship with food is a healthy one. Experts believe that the greater part of individuals who are overweight or obese have some level of food addiction. However, anyone of all ages and size can have this issue.

2) Know your staples from your treats. Our brains are fixed to search out the tasty reward of natural carbs like berries from a bramble or veggies from the ground. We enjoy healthy fats from avocados, olive oil, and fish and incline meats. Our brains drive us to forage around to find these foods with the goal that we have snappy vitality (from carbs) and long-lasting fuel (from fat). These natural entire foods have sustained us since the beginning of time. Our brains were acclimated to the taste of these prizes. From time to time, we'd appreciate a treat that contained more natural sugar (grapes) or fat (dairy or meat). This blend of staples and treats became our natural adjust of healthy supplements. Flash-forward, and now we have makers creating "hyperpalatable" foods loaded with sugar, fat, and salt. What's more, because they are ubiquitous, shoddy, and easily available, less individuals cook. Snatch and go is presently the approach.

3) Rein in your reward focus. At the point when hyperpalatables rival natural foods, your brain's reward focus, which secretes the pleasure concoction dopamine, gets seized. Insulin levels go up and push you to need to an ever increasing extent. Abruptly, that bowl of crisp berries can't contend with the über prizes of a Pop–Tart or a chocolate–coated breakfast bar. An occasional treat, for example, a birthday dessert, also prompts to a dopamine surge, but then your brain settles down to more ordinary levels of dopamine. But when you can get your hands on hyperpalatable foods day in and day out and you begin the day with that sugary/fatty/salty pastry and grande sugary coffee drink, you wind up with an unending craving for additional.

5) Recognize the "False Fix." After constant introduction and consumption of these hyperpalatables, which I allude to as "False Fixes" in The Hunger Fix, your brain really changes. The brain cannot tolerate this level of hyperstimulation. Accordingly, it decreases the number of dopamine receptors so that you no longer feel it as overstimulation. That's the uplifting news. The awful news is that by doing this, your common serving of food is no longer as rewarding. You find yourself not feeling as pleased and satisfied. You know the final product. Not satisfied, you wind up with second and third and fourth portions, packing on weight along the way.

But hold up, there's additional: in the meantime your reward focus is being commandeered, the brain's CEO, the prefrontal cortex (tap your forehead and that's where the PFC is located), is becoming harmed and impeded. The PFC can no longer help you rein in driving forces or remain focused and watchful. That's the reason, when someone is in all out addictive mode, moderation is a disputable issue. Revolutionary and groundbreaking new reviews supported by the National Institutes of Health subsidized have shown that the brain scans of food addicts show an indistinguishable changes and harm from those of a cocaine client. Furthermore, for your information, inquire about also shows that table sugar (sucrose) is more addictive than cocaine.

Good, what's the solution? Science–based detox and recovery from the foods and beverages that you know are causing you to lose control and overeat.

6) Know your adversary. Make a rundown the greater part of your False Fix foods that you know will lead you to feel crazy and overeat. As you get ready to detox, check out you and inventory the persons, places, and things that empower your food addiction. This isn't just about switching up False Fix foods for Healthy Fixes. It's also about examining your whole lifestyle so you can make new, healthier decisions to support your recovery. You're not going to change everything overnight, so you'll begin with

little but effective strides to guarantee sustainable, long–term achievement.

7) Remember these words: MIND, MOUTH, MUSCLE. That will help you sort out how you'll detox and recover.

MIND: Reclaim your brain. A strong PFC is totally required to repair and recover your reward focus. What's more, you can repair your PFC with supernatural meditation and mindfulness. The key is to practice them every day to stimulate new brain cell formation and to repair harm. When you meditate you cause genuine brain changes to help repair and reinforce brain cells.

MOUTH: Get high... naturally. Accomplish a natural "high" from entire foods that increase dopamine production naturally. Specific foods watermelon, spinach, avocados, tofu, and sesame seeds, to give some examples perform enchantment and restore typical reward responses for natural foods. Also, utilize intense protein and fiber combinations carrots and hummus, nut or almond butter and apple cuts, for instance that satisfy and stop the inclination to spend too much on sugary/fatty/salty foods.

MUSCLE: Every progression you take during the day stimulates brain development, including your PFC, which translates to a greater, stronger, more focused brain. Furthermore, one of the mottos of The Hunger Fix is BIG BRAIN, SMALL WAIST. You'll settle on more astute decisions and shed additional weight if your brain is healthy. Look into has also shown that consistent physical movement will also keep you more settled and decrease the shot of backslide. All you need is standard moderate practice to make this work. Walking is the easiest approach for a great many people. Doing it outdoors and stepping up the pace when you can upgrades the whole experience and results. I'm not talking marathons here, people. Simply getting up and moving.

Fast food has become a common staple in the diet of many individuals. Late controversy over how unhealthy fast food is has driven numerous individuals to begin looking for effective approaches to get out from under their fast food propensities and choose healthier feast options. Notwithstanding why you choose fast food, understand that you can get out from under the propensity. Following these tips can help you decrease your fast food consumption and may control you towards a healthier method for eating.

Method1

Understanding Food Addiction

1. Gather food addiction assets. If you genuinely feel like you have a food addiction, it'll be useful to completely understand what food addiction it is and how it affects your life.

•Food addiction can be a difficult problem. High sugar and high fat foods are to a great degree palatable. Whenever eaten, they trigger the release of dopamine to the brain's reward focus. This triggers the yearning to eat a greater amount of that food and to come back to it again.

•People with Binge–eating Disorder feel a compulsion to eat bizarrely a lot of food in a brief period of time.They may feel nauseated by their eating propensities but can't control them. If you feel constrained to eat substantial quantities of fast food, regardless of the possibility that you feel awful afterward, consider seeing a mental health professional about the likelihood of Binge–eating Disorder. It's exceedingly treatable.

•Spend some time researching food addiction online. There are an assortment of sources online that might be ready to help you take in more about your eating propensities.

•Purchase or look at a library book on food addiction. Invest some energy reading and researching about food addictions.

2. Record your problems with food. Seeing your food addiction issues recorded can make them all the more genuine to you. Include how often you eat fast food, your feelings or cravings around fast food and how hard you think it'll be to surrender it.

• To help you understand the seriousness of your food addiction, ask yourself if you are frail around fast food or what emotions or situations make you pine for fast food.

• Also rate your feelings of addiction from 1 to 10 (one being frail and 10 being immensely strong). The rating may change with your emotions but it can give you insight into times, occasions or individuals that influence your rating.

• Write down all the specific sorts of food that you feel dependent on. Is it only fast food? Then again does your addiction include "garbage foods" like candy, potato chips or pop?

3. Roll out a lifestyle improvement, don't begin a diet. Diets, in the traditional sense are not sustainable long term plans, particularly not for a food addiction.

• People surrender, stop purchasing the diet items or get exhausted and stop. Intend to roll out a lifestyle improvement around your food addiction and don't simply receive a diet.

•Write up a food plan that does not include fast food or garbage food. Ensure you plan for appropriate portion sizes and snacks so you don't become too ravenous at any point during the day.

•Remove "trigger" foods from your home if your addiction includes other garbage foods in addition to fast food. If you are as yet eating a lot of fat and sugar (enter ingredients in fast food) at home, it will be harder to break your addiction to fast food.

Method2

Eliminating Fast Food

1. Pack healthy suppers and snacks. Having a healthy feast or snack accessible is a great approach to decrease the measure of fast food you consume. Instead of going out to eat, you as of now have your healthy feast arranged and prepared to–go.

•Purchase a little lunch box or cooler if fundamental. This is a great approach to stay away from a stop at a fast food place. Keeping it stocked with healthy options like yogurt, crisp natural products or carrots and hummus can help you adhere to your planned dinner or to control your yearning until you can return home for your feast.

•Keep healthy, convenient snacks, for example, portioned nuts or organic product in your satchel, briefcase or car.

•Make beyond any doubt to eat throughout the day. Don't skip suppers. Snatch a healthy snack if you're feeling hungry. When you are exceptionally eager, will probably settle on terrible food decisions.

2. Stop drinking pop. For some individuals, this may end up being the greatest test. Attempt to stay away from all sodas. Indeed, even diet sodas ought to be minimized in your diet. Diet sodas may confuse your body into feeling hungry notwithstanding when you don't have to eat.

•Aim for 64 oz of clear, without sugar fluids every day. You can attempt water, water seasoned with herbs and natural product, unsweetened frosted tea or unsweetened decaf coffee.

•If this progression turns out to be difficult, begin off slowly. Begin decreasing the measure of pop you consume by replacing a couple drinks here and there with a healthier option (like water or unsweetened tea). Continue substituting other drinks for your pop until you can eliminate pop altogether.

3. Drive a different course. Sometimes simply driving past (or knowing you'll pass) your most loved fast food place is sufficient to make you pull over. Driving a different course to work or on your way home may help get you out of the routine of stopping for fast food.

•Check out an online guide. Many projects allow you to put in your starting and ending location and give you an assortment of course options.

•If you can't bypass a fast food place, take a stab at putting up a note in your car with an idealistic sentence. "You can do it!" or "Concentrate on your objective!" are great phrases that can keep you driving right on by.

4. Work out the upsides of eliminating fast food. Giving up fast food won't not be easy. However, having a rundown of positive thoughts to audit

when a strong craving hits, can be a useful asset to help you overcome the drive through path.

> •Take 60 minutes (this could be a piece of your activities in a diary) and work out a rundown of the considerable number of favorable circumstances of giving up fast food. Positive thoughts could include weight reduction, saving money, increased vitality or better health.

> •Keep a duplicate of your positive thoughts in your tote or wallet, car or at work. Allude to it at whatever point you have a craving for a fast food dinner.

As you continue to avoid fast food, expound on your advance and include the positive occasions you've seen about your lifestyle, health and diet. This will help extend that rundown.1.

5. Go to healthier restaurants. Going out for lunch is a common workplace movement. You can enjoy a reprieve and appreciate 30 to a hour from your work area. If you and your coworkers regularly stop by a fast food restaurant, propose something healthier.

> •Research restaurants that are near your workplace. Look at their menus and check whether these eventual a

better option for you and your partners.

•Let your coworkers know you're trying to drop your fast food propensity. You never know, they might need to join you! Letting individuals around you think about your objectives allows them to support you, rather than be an awful influence.

•Agree to a lunch out only one time seven days. If companions are unwilling to budge on lunch time options, only go out once per week. This can help minimize your temptations.

Method3

Planning a Strategy

1. Work out practical objectives. Giving yourself a long–term objective to work towards can help ease you out of your fast food propensity. Ensure you set a practical and specific objective that you can accomplish over time.

•Set littler objectives along the route to your long–term one. Maybe you begin by skipping the drive through on Mondays or plan to eat breakfast at home. Trying to handle various objectives at once can be difficult.

•Being sensible with objective setting is vital. If you feel that failing to have fast food again is not practical, set a breaking point to how much you can have. Maybe you allow yourself a fast food feast once per month.

•Track the advance of your objective overtime. This can help motivate you and keep you on track towards your long–term objective.

2. Purchase a diary or scratch pad. Utilize your diary to take note of your dinners and snacks for a couple days (in a perfect world a couple week days and a couple ends of the week). This will give you insight into how much and how often you're consuming fast food.

•Also note situations that make you choose fast food regularly. For example, do you experience the drive–through on the best approach to work for breakfast? On the other hand do you have a long drive home and stop by for a snappy and easy dinner?

•Take note of any temperaments or emotions that may trigger you to eat or long for fast food. You may see numerous days you don't consume fast food. It may happen all the more often when you're focused, irate or frustrated. Understanding your connection between food and disposition can help give you some insight into your fast food propensity.

•Don't have sufficient energy to diary? Download a food diary application for an on–the–go version of your food diary. Having the application open on your phone can make it a tad bit easier.

•Think about why you make the fast food stops. Trying to identify the underlying reason for your fast food addiction is a critical stride in breaking the propensity.

•Note how you feel after eating fast food. You may feel remorseful, liable, or ashamed. If you see negative feelings and record them, you can reference them later on before deciding to get fast food. Remembering how awful you feel after eating it might help you keep away from it.

3. Number the calories. If you haven't represented the calories you're consuming in fast food suppers,

you may be astounded at how much you're really consuming. Take a day and count up every one of the calories of your run of the mill fast food dinner. The number may be sufficient to give you the motivation to drop the propensity.

•Try figuring out how far you'd need to run or bicycle to smolder off that dinner. It more often than not takes a considerable measure of practice to blaze off the calories from a fast food dinner. For example, you need to bicycle an entire hour at a rapid to smolder about 800 calories, that's a large portion of a pizza...

•Compare the calories in your fast food dinner to a comparative suppers that you could make yourself at home. It'll help you understand what number more calories you get from fast food.

4. Track the expenses of your fast food propensity. One of the benefits of fast food is that it can be truly shabby – particularly with menu things that are $1.00 or less. Indeed, even with these low prices, fast food can in any case include.

•Keep your receipts and include how much money you spend in one week. It may be more than you think.

•Give yourself $10 or $20 in cash and perceive how long that lasts you throughout the week. It's easy to swipe a credit or plastic. Cash is sometimes harder to part with.

5. Work out a week by week dinner plan. Having a set supper plan in place may help keep you to remain composed and focused throughout the week. You won't be wondering what you're making for dinner or bringing for lunch – it's been determined as of now!

•Take a hour or two during your available time to work out your feast plan. Try to include breakfast and snacks for every day too.

•Consider including recipes or supper ideas for fast, easy–to–plan dinners to help you with your bustling lifestyle.

•After your feast plan is finished, review the corresponding basic supply list. You'll be ready to purchase only what you require.

6. Go shopping for food. Having healthy food on hand is vital to giving up fast food. Shop week by week for suppers and snacks so you generally have another, healthier option prepared to–go.

•Stock up on incline protein, natural products, vegetables, entire grains and low–fat dairy items.

•Purchase prepared to–eat items that oblige practically no cooking and can be eaten on–the–go. Examples include entire natural products (like an apple or banana), individual yogurts, – washed and cut plates of mixed greens or vegetables or precooked incline protein (like barbecued chicken fingers).

Method4

Implementing Coping Strategies

1. Build a support network. Any adjustment in diet can be difficult – particularly if you're giving up a propensity that feels like a food addiction. Having a support group can help motivate you and empower you as you roll out difficult improvements. Thinks about have shown that many individuals stay with positive changes longer if they have a support group.

•Ask relatives, companions or coworkers to support you. In addition, you can check whether anyone might want to join you on your adventure to surrender fast food.

•Research online support groups and forums that you can sign on throughout the day. It's a great approach to have support at whatever time of the day.

2. Converse with an enlisted dietitian and an authorized therapist. These health and nutrition experts can assume a key part in helping you understand and overcome your fast food propensity. They have the training to help you drop the fast food propensity, help you plan healthier dinners in addition to giving you coping systems to manage your food addiction.

•Ask a dietitian for help with feast planning, cooking abilities or basic nutrition information so you have the right stuff important to drop your fast food propensity.

•Discuss with an authorized therapist about your food addiction and any emotional eating issues that have come up.

•Check with your essential care or other doctor for a referral to an enlisted dietitian or authorized therapist. They may know or work with someone locally.

3. Work out a rundown of self–soothing exercises. When you're pushed or a fast food craving hits hard, it's vital to have a rundown of exercises that you can do to occupy yourself and quiet down. Have these handy when a craving hits.

•Try engaging in mentally and physically dynamic things. For example: taking a walk, cleaning out your garbage drawer, calling a companion or relative, keeping a diary or reading a decent book.

•Sleeping longer or getting lost in TV may not improve you feel. You're not addressing the issue at hand. Instead, it's being disregarded or rested through.

•Try to avoid drinking mixed beverages. Drinking liquor is never an appropriate coping component for addiction.

•Write down your feelings. Understand that scratch pad or diary out and record your feelings and how they are affecting your cravings or feelings of yearning.

•Keeping a diary can help you unmistakably identify your situation and have the effect between emotional eating and physical appetite.

•A diary can also act like a mental release allowing you to spill out every one of your emotions and feelings onto paper.

4. Meditate. Thinks about have shown that even a couple of minutes of meditation can quiet your mind, help you feel more focused and assist you in overcoming addiction. This can be an easy approach to help ease your mind.

•Start with only 5 to 10 minutes a day – particularly if you've never attempted meditation.

•Check online with the expectation of complimentary sound guided meditations. These can help you ease yourself into meditation by following the tender orders of a guide.

•Try dynamic meditation which allows you to concentrate on a little question – a stone, a natural product or a gem. This can help give your mind some occupation while you attempt to remain in the present.

5. Stock your wash room, refrigerator and cooler with healthy foods. Continuously keep a stock of healthy things at home. This will allow you to cook

nutritious suppers without having to stop at the store on your way home.

•Having a very much stocked home may help alleviate the worry around cooking or getting a dinner on the table. You'll as of now be set up with the basics of a dinner.

•Pantry staples can include beans, canned vegetables with no salt included, canned fish, entire grains (like brown rice or entire wheat pasta) and nuts.

•Freezer staples can include solidified protein (like chicken or fish), solidified vegetables and organic product, solidified cooked entire grains (like brown rice or quinoa) and low-calorie solidified suppers (for a night that cooking isn't an option).

•Refrigerator staples can include washed and cut foods grown from the ground, low-fat dressings and sauces, eggs, low-fat yogurt and cheddar and cooked proteins (like barbecued chicken breasts).

6. Get ready new recipes. Whether you you're in a recipe trench or need some help coming up with healthy suppers, trying new recipes is a great

approach to investigate an assortment of different healthy foods. Attempt one or two new recipes every week.

•Need recipe ideas? Take a stab at purchasing a healthy eating cookbook, looking up healthy eat web journals online or asking companions or family for new recipes to attempt.

•If you're short on time, scan for recipes that require minimal cooking and preparation. Ordinarily, you can simply assemble your feast instead of preparing everything from scratch.

7. Recreate your fast food top choices at home. Burgers and fries or chicken strips are flavorful – that's the reason it's hard to bring an end to a fast food propensity. Have a go at making your top picks at home with healthier cooking techniques. This will help you to "indulge" but with a much healthier option.

•If you cherish fries, have a go at baking them at home. Cut sweet potatoes also make a great french sear alternative. Plus they have a lot of vitamins and minerals!

•Bread chicken with smashed cornflakes or saltines and bake for a crunchy, low-calorie version of seared chicken or chicken strips.

•Research some recipes online for your top choices. You'll find some great ideas and an assortment of recipes for healthier versions of common fast food dinners. Take a stab at searching for "fast food swaps" to find healthier substitutes for your most loved fast food options.

Method5

Eating Healthy at Fast Food Restaurants

1. Perused online menus. Any restaurant with over 20 locations is legally required to have an online menu and a menu in store that contains the majority of the nutrition information. Audit the menu for options that are lower in calorie and lower in fat.

•Plan your dinner option before going out to eat. This will help keep you from temptations by reviewing the menu or hearing what others are ordering.

•Some places even have "feast calculators" that will allow you to choose different options for your dinner and gives the calorie and other nutrition information for you.

2. Choose barbecued options over browned. Broiled foods commonly contain more calories and fat contrasted with barbecued things.

> •Go for a barbecued chicken sandwich or flame broiled chicken strips instead of fricasseed chicken.

3. Maintain a strategic distance from the combo suppers. The calorie number can get quite high when you get a combination feast – fries, sandwich and drink. Simply purchase the sandwich instead for a lower calorie check.

> •Choose things from the "individually" menu (one after another) to stay away from the option of the combination supper.

> •Refuse the upgrade for a "super–estimate" or greater portion.

4. Purchase a healthier option. Many fast food restaurants have been responding to consumers wishes for healthier options. They even have unique "healthier" menus that can guide you toward a lower calorie dinner.

> •Try a serving of mixed greens with flame broiled chicken or a barbecued chicken wrap. Utilize a little portion of light dressing or dipping sauce to help keep the calories lower.

•If you're stopping by for breakfast, attempt oatmeal, yogurt with natural product or a breakfast sandwich with an egg white and cheddar.

•Choose a sandwich with a side of natural product or a vegetable side instead of the run of the mill french fries.Addiction does not generally need to involve an addictive substance or drug, as the term can be used to describe an unreasonable behavior, for example, habitual eating. While there are different schools of thought and the scientific literature in the region of food addiction is still in the beginning stages, numerous experts believe that addiction to food truly isn't about the food.

To elaborate further, foods don't have addictive properties that make someone rely on upon them, unlike compound substances. Food addiction has more to do with how a person behaves around food, what they think about food, and the way propensities are formed with food. The propensities are the genuine wellspring of the addiction.

Food can become an approach to adapt to emotional matters, and the repetition of this coping instrument can breed an addiction. By using food as a way to manage anxiety, stress, sorrow, and so forth, the body becomes conditioned to ache for that procedure to feel help.

Individuals often associate pleasure with foods that contain fat, sugar and salt. As innocent as it might appear, this begins at a youthful age when candy and pop are given as a "treat" or "reward" for good behavior, grades or a celebration. Explore examines have shown the reward centers of the brain to light up and release dopamine when pleasurable foods are consumed. Could this be that we've conditioned our bodies to respond this way?

The Slippery Slope of Food Addiction

Someone doesn't simply conclude that he or she needs to feel wild with food. It's often a slippery slant that leads a person into an addiction with food. Below are some of the warning signs and common qualities among individuals suffering from a food addiction:

- Changes in state of mind

- Labeling food as "great" and "terrible"

- Restrictive dieting

- Eating in secret or sneaking food

- Feeling crazy with food

- Rewarding/treating yourself with food

- Thinking about food constantly

- Feeling unsatisfied even after feast times

- Weight fluctuations as well as difficulty managing weight

- Body dissatisfaction

- Feeling nauseated, liable or upset after eating

- Feeling focused or tension that is only mitigated by eating

How To Overcome Food Addiction

Recovering from a food addiction is a procedure, and one that merits taking to find flexibility from food. Taking the power over from food often requires a group approach keeping in mind the end goal to accomplish a full recovery. Here are a couple ventures to take to help someone recovering from food addiction:

1.Develop a Healthy Relationship with Food. In traditional 12–stage addiction–based recovery models, addicts are tested to remain abstinent for healing. However, with food addiction, one can't just abstain by not eating, as food is basic to life. Along these lines someone suffering with food addiction must figure out how to eat properly again by establishing a healthy relationship with food.

2.Set Boundaries with Unsafe Foods. Ordinarily, trigger or "dangerous" foods are expelled from the diet and limits are set so that managing these foods in a healthier manner can be relearned. If someone binges on dessert when he or she is focused on, it's best not to keep it in the house. Eliminating the temptation until he or she can eat frozen yogurt again in an adjusted manner is a sheltered option.

3.Follow a Structured Meal Plan. A person suffering from an unhealthy relationship with food can get on the right track to recovery by following a supper plan and typical eating pattern. This helps the person set safe limits with food, and feel satisfied so that there is not a physiological need to eat. It's additionally tempting to be wild with food when there is physical deprivation.

4.Learn Healthy Coping Strategies. Deliver reasons for turning to food to adapt. Identify healthier coping systems and strategies so one can begin learning healthier method for dealing with emotions.

5.Seek Professional Advice. Beating a food addiction is a procedure and does not occur without any forethought; it often needs to involve an enrolled dietitian and authorized therapist that have practical experience in the region of disordered eating. These professionals will help a person suffering from food addiction implement appropriate strategies, and give responsibility and sound advice.

Recovery from a food addiction is achievable. If you or a friend or family member is suffering, share this , give reassurance, and urge him or her to find professional support.

Chapter 19
Techniques to Eliminate Food Addictions

At the point when a large portion of us think of food addiction, we tend to picture outrageous cases like My 600 lb Life on TLC, which is incompletely because we associate the expression "addiction" with substantial substance mishandle like drugs and liquor. This makes it easy to assume that someone suffering from a food addiction must measure an outrageous sum because they've gone overboard with their eating propensities.

Unfortunately, this simply isn't the case.

Like the recently coined term, Dad Bod, there's another expression called being Skinny Fat. This happens when a person is really a healthy weight, but makes due on an unhealthy diet and confines calories in an effort to combat their poor food decisions so they don't gain any weight.

But these are quite recently some examples of food addiction. The reality of the situation is that a hefty portion of us are battling our own food addictions and we may not understand it.

With that stated, it's an ideal opportunity to take in more.

What Is A Food Addiction?

lady staring food addictionAlthough 'food addiction' is genuine and genuine, there's no official definition of what it is precisely. On top of that, like any addiction, it can go up against many forms ranging from an obsession with calorie counting or restricting your food intake to downright overeating. The term can also be used when certain foods, like garbage food, really make you be dependent.

Thus, for the reason for this , we'll keep it straightforward and say that a food addiction can be anything from an obsession with food, to uncontrollable desires for certain foods that prompt to overeating. What's more, the overeating in this case does not really mean you eat too numerous calories, rather, it can imply that you're overeating the wrong sorts of food, as in the case with being Skinny Fat.

You could truly be dependent on foods, for example, you're morning coffee or late night desserts. Without those staples in your routine, you may find yourself bad tempered or unhappy. If that's the case, you may have a food addiction on your hands.

Since the definition is somewhat unclear, here are a couple of things to watch out for.

According to Food Addicts these are:

Do you find that certain foods give you that 'I can't simply eat one' feeling?

Is it accurate to say that you are constantly thinking about food or when and where your next supper will originate from?

Do you eat another way when you are home alone versus out with companions?

Do you eat extensive quantities of food in one sitting instead of spacing out littler suppers?

Is it true that you are someone who snacks throughout the day and never really feels full?

Do you fast or limit your calorie intake drastically in an effort to counteract weight gain?

Do you eat when you're exhausted and not really ravenous?

Have you wanted to overexercise in an attempt to offset a terrible eating routine?

Is it accurate to say that you are over the top about what number calories you take in versus what number you blaze?

Do you feel liable or ashamed when you eat an "awful" dinner?

Have you surrendered or felt miserable that weight reduction is unattainable for you?

I need to point out that these are not by any means the only questions you ought to be asking yourself if you think you could have a genuine food addiction.

What I've attempted to show you here is that a food addiction can be more common than you think.

But what makes this an addiction?

The Addiction Behind Food Addiction

lady enjoying strawberriesWe can be dependent on food thanks to the way that certain foods can trigger your brain to respond in a comparative manner that drugs and liquor can.

Have you ever wondered why a smoker can't simply up and quit cigarettes despite the several warnings and plugs touting that smoking causes cancer?

Drugs and liquor cause a disruption in your brain's typical science adjust, and unfortunately, some foods can have that same effect.

Here's how it works.

Our brains have been wired to respond to our general surroundings. For example, when you touch something hot, your brain sends a flag to move your hand so you're not left with a blaze.

In the case of drugs and food addiction, 'feel great' flags in the form of dopamine – a neurotransmitter responsible for sending out messages from our brain to our nerves – surges our brains when we 'utilize', whether that's through food or drugs. This surge of positive sentiments is like having natural morphine flowing through your veins. It can give you an euphoric feeling that leaves you without a care on the planet.The problem is, because we experience this procedure in the form of a 'surge', the feeling is fleeting. Once the surge is gone, you're left in a 'crash–like' state wanting more. This is what causes drug addicts to continue using, and the same goes for food addicts.

I needed to wonder, what is it that makes certain foods so addictive?

That is to say, have you ever attempted to eat only one Girl Scout treat? It's practically inconceivable, at least for me.

I believe that the two greatest guilty parties making us debilitated are included sugars and food added substances.

Here are the greatest food added substances to watch out for. You'll find these ingredients recorded right on the nutrition labels of some of the most common garbage food.

Food Additives Can Make You Addicted To Food

The reason a large portion of us can't simply eat one potato chip or one treat is thanks to some extent to the food added substances that are found in our ordinary foods. One of the most exceedingly terrible offenders is monosodium glutamate, also known as MSG.

Monosodium glutamate, MSG

noodles MSGMany individuals know about MSG because of their nearby Chinese food take out restaurants, but that's by all account not the only place it's hiding. It's a little ingredient added to food as a method for enhancing flavor.

Cerebral pains

Gentle temperament changes

Tingling

Heart palpitations

Distinctive or strange dreams

Burning sensations

Snugness in the trunk

Indeed, even asthma like symptoms

The greater part of that is conceivable from something as little as a sack of potato chips.

But, that's not all.

According to a report from Fox News, inquire about conducted on creatures found that MSG can trigger a 40% increase in hunger. The review also stated: "Individuals who consume the most MSG are nearly three circumstances more prone to be overweight than the individuals who don't eat it by any means".

MSG is what's responsible for that 'I can't simply eat one' feeling. You know, the one you get when your arm is mostly down the tube of a Pringles can. You can thank MSG that.

This tiny ingredient confuses your body by shutting down the hormone leptin, which is responsible for telling your brain that you're full. The final product: you can't stop eating.

Also, this transforms into an endless loop whereby the more MSG you eat, the more you will want foods that make them set, the perfect stage for an unsuspecting food addiction.

But MSG isn't the only one to fault. High fructose corn syrup (HFCS) is also to blame.

High fructose corn syrup

corn syrupRemember those tasty Girl Scout treats I mentioned before? Indeed, HFCS might be the reason you can't eat only one.

I often find that there's some confusion regarding HFCS because of the current dispatch of advertisements supported by the corn industry (Yes that's right) that advance it being protected, healthy, and bravo.

So what precisely is high fructose corn syrup?

To put it plainly, HFCS is a corn syrup that's been scientifically engineered and contains added compounds to make it taste sweeter than traditional corn syrups.

It's used as a modest approach to make foods taste sweeter and you'll find it in the majority of your handled "desserts" available, including our beloved Girl Scout treats.

The problem is, unlike traditional sugar, your body does not understand how to prepare the Frankenstein ingredient so it winds up getting stored as fat.

A group of researchers at Princeton University concentrated the effects of HFCS on rats and the outcomes were astonishing. "Rats with access to high fructose corn syrup gained significantly more weight than those with access to table sugar, notwithstanding when their overall caloric intake was the same".

The exploration also demonstrated that, "in addition to causing significant weight gain in lab creatures, long term consumption of high fructose corn syrup prompted to irregular increases in muscle to fat quotients, particularly in the abdomen".

As if that wasn't sufficient, this hurtful added substance also increases your cravings for high fat foods, creating an endless loop that can transform into a food addiction.

In one review, researchers thought about the effects of fructose, the sugar found in HFCS, to glucose, or traditional table sugar.

Members were given a cherry enhanced drink that either contained 2.5 oz of fructose or glucose. The individuals examined were given a scale to rate how hungry they were preceding drinking the beverage.

Members were then shown pictures of unhealthy foods and asked whether they would want to eat that food now or save it in return for a monetary honor one month later.

The outcome: the individuals who consumed the fructose drink will probably choose the fatty foods instead of waiting for the reward. Researchers could conclude that the fructose corn syrups really increase your cravings for fatty foods.

Like MSG, HFCS is a subtle little ingredient that could be causing our food addictions or making them more awful.

So if MSG and HFCS are both added substances used to improve foods taste, what about the artificial sweeteners used to make foods taste sweeter without using any calories?

How would they affect our health?

Artificial sweeteners

aspartame tabletsWith the ascent of low calorie diets came the need drinks that tasted as great as their original versions, but contain zero sugars or calories.

Introducing artificial sweeteners.

The most common ones are:

Acesulfame potassium

Aspartame (what you'd find in the blue Equal parcels)

High fructose corn syrup

Neotame (discovered predominantly in zero calorie drinks)

Saccharin (what you'd find in pink Sweet'N Low bundles)

Sucralose (found in Splenda bundles)

Sugar alcohols, for example, sorbitol, xylitol, mannitol, and erythritol

These terrible young men can be as much as 40 to 700 circumstances sweeter than standard sugar without any of the calories!

In principle, artificial sweeteners sound great; they're zero calorie season helps. But, although you're saving on calories, you could in any case wind up gaining weight according to a compilation of studies distributed in the US National Library of Medicine.The American Cancer Society conducted a review in the 1980s on the effects of artificial sweeteners on 78,694 women. The individuals who consumed the artificial sweeteners showed a 7.1% increase in weight.

At this point you might be wondering how artificial sweeteners make you gain weight and become dependent, and that's a reasonable question.

These toxic sweeteners:

Stimulate your hunger

Increase cravings for carbohydrates

Energize fat storage

As you can see, artificial sweeteners are yet another contributor to the food addiction cycle.

One of my most loved books by big name personal trainer Jackie Warner, This is Why You're Fat and How to Get Thin Forever, stresses that sugars are to be faulted for our food addiction.

All things considered, Jackie Warner believes that additional sugar is in too numerous foods found in our present diet.

Included sugars

refined sugar cubesI showed you in this that shrouded sugars are everywhere, so I couldn't concur more with Warner. I've even shown you how to dodge the abundance sugars in this .

The point is, the point at which we consume sugars, we wind up craving them significantly more throughout the day.

So if you begin your morning with a decent, enhanced coffee and your sweetener is a sugar bound flavor or you include your own artificial sweetener bundles, you're going to wind up craving sugar and carbohydrates for whatever is left of the day.

This is what makes us dependent. That feeling of wondering about where our 'next settle' is makes it hard for us to state no to garbage food. Our "settle" is snacking on or eating things we know aren't precisely healthy for us, but pine for in any case.

Since you know why we're dependent, we should discuss how to break the addiction.

How To Cut Your Food Addiction

1. Don't simply take a gander at calorie numbers, read ingredient labels

lady reading ingredientsIf losing weight and living healthy are your objectives, don't simply stop at the measure of calories in food. Look at the ingredients too. Check whether you can spot any of the ingredients I've recorded in today's post. If you can, it's a great opportunity to dump that item and never think back.

2. Skip zero calorie options

opening diet cokeFrom this point forward, I trust that you'll forgo anything labeled as zero calories or zero sugars. Whether that's a drink, snack, or plate of mixed greens dressing, a significant number of these foods are using unhealthy artificial sweeteners that could be leaving you more regrettable off than when you began.

Maintain a strategic distance from these terrible young men at all expenses to break the cycle of addiction.

3. Begin making healthier swaps

potatoes chips saltTry making healthier swaps and slowly transition out of eating foods that contain the ingredients I've recorded here.

So if potato chips are your thing, search for assortments that don't contain MSG so you're ready to satisfy your salty craving without overdoing it. Obviously, regardless you'll have to practice portion control regardless of the possibility that the chips don't contain MSG.

4. Don't begin your day with enhanced coffee

green tea potI'm beyond any doubt large portions of you will hate me for this one, but I ask you to stop starting your day on the wrong foot by drinking coffee with included flavors and flavors. Swap out your morning mix for green tea instead.

By consuming sugar filled coffees at an opportune time, you're only setting yourself up for a day loaded with cravings and unhealthy snacking.

5. Keep away from included sugars at whatever point conceivable

holding sugar cubesDon't assume that your appetizing dinner is free from sugars. Look at my rundown of foods that contain high measures of sugar and maintain a strategic distance from them at all expenses. Some of them may astound you.

6. Connect with an expert

happy nutritionistEnding your food addiction can be similarly as hard as quitting liquor or drugs, and sometimes, you may require assistance from a professional. That's alright. The sooner you can get help, the sooner you can begin living healthier.

Find a neighborhood nutritionist or therapist in your general vicinity who has some expertise in food addiction and let him realize what foods you have a tendency to pine for additional. He might be your best bet for getting help.

Since you know a food addiction can transpire at whatever time, I trust you'll reconsider some of the decisions you might be making. If you're eating foods with added substances, for example, MSG or HFCS, you could be putting a great deal more at hazard than simply your waistline.

Chapter 20
A Week of Meals to Break Your Junk Food Addiction

I am dependent on unhealthy food. Sometimes I escape with it because I rehearse Brazilian jiu jitsu, which smolders a lot of calories. But during injury rehabilitation, the weight gain happens rapidly. I'm working on getting free of this unhealthy reliance. Furthermore, I'm using a strategy from the last time I quit doing something stupid effectively.

When I was thirteen, I began smoking. I smoked until I was 25 and chose I was too old to continue. I assumed I would settle down and have a family, and I would not like to be dependent on cigarettes when it came time to get pregnant. Since I am forty, I live alone with three cats. Although I never got pregnant, quitting the cigarettes was clearly the best decision for my health.

Continuous Change for Lasting Effects

The smoking strategy was straightforward. Every day I had my first cigarette of the day fifteen minutes later than the day preceding. So on the very beginning, my first cigarette was at 8:30am, the following day, 8:45, et cetera. If I sat tight until my booked time for the main cigarette, I could smoke as much as I needed afterwards. If I smoked before my booked time, I couldn't smoke at all for whatever is left of the day. By the time I got to three months, I was no longer dependent on cigarettes, and I haven't smoked routinely since.

So how can we apply that strategy to our diets? It's about the steady change. For me, it's not about throwing the majority of my garbage food away and entirely adhering to my new diet. It's not about beginning with a painful detox or wash down (which are absurd, by the way). I was never ready to stop smoking or do anything else "without any weaning period." I was ready to stop because of two reasons:

1.It was essential to me to stop for the sole purpose of being healthy for future objectives.

2.I never felt denied during the quitting procedure.

Week by week Meal Plan for Athletes

So here I am nearing the finish of recovery for a back injury I sustained in August of last year, and I am slowly but most likely losing the weight I gained. For your purpose and mine, I have built up a week after week dinner plan, finish with recipes, and a definite basic supply list. This plan is my objective for a perfect week of eating.

Supplements

Supplements assist us with recovery and health. The dominant part of our nutrition originates from genuine food. Based on my examination, I have settled on the following supplements to improve my health and performance:

Day by day Supplements:

- Krill Oil, Fish Oil, Flax Seed Oil or Micro green growth oil totaling EPA 2400mg and DPA 1800mg

- Vitimin D3: 4000iu

- Magnesium Citrate: 400mg (or make this smoothie)

- Creatine: 5mg

- Green Tea: 1–2 cups

- Black Tea: 1–2 cups

During + Post Training:

- BCAAs (during training)

- Protein + Dextrose (post–training). This ought to be consumed rapidly, rather than tasted. I take one scoop of protein and about 40g of dextrose.

- Chamomile Tea: I fill a Thermos before training and drink it on my path home to quiet my framework after training and plan for rest. Remember, rest is the most imperative thing you can accomplish for your health. Be certain to get eight hours a night.A Perfect Week of Meals

In a perfect training week, I train Brazilian jiu jitsu three days a week and do two days of quality and conditioning. I take one night off each week and walk a normal of 10,000 stages a day, according to my Jawbone movement tracker.

My supper planning approach:

•Sunday evening I prepare suppers for the following week.

•I set up my omelet filling for a few days and my suppers for Sunday night, Monday, and Tuesday until lunch.

•Tuesday night, I cook supper and dinners for Wednesday and Thursday lunch.

•Thursday night, I cook supper and lunch for Friday

•For whatever is left of the end of the week I am ready to cook as required.

Learn Patience and Consistency

Developing this dinner plan has been a slow procedure. In the beginning, I cooked one or two suppers from my Precision Nutrition cookbook per week. Whatever remains of the time, I ate the way I ordinarily would have. In the long run, I cooked three, then four suppers that were based on the cookbook. I began enjoying these healthy suppers more than the food I used to eat.

After gradually changing my diet over a while, I anticipate eating these healthy dinners consistently and I appreciate experimenting with different recipes. I feel better, and I'm starting to look better. Once I'm back on the mats at full limit, I know I'll perform better. I trust this dinner plan will be a helpful tool for you as well.

Chapter 21
Mind Tricks to Beat Your Food Addiction and Stop Emotional Eating

Food is a Drug

Food is a drug. This is an unquestionable actuality.

You can become physiologically dependent, like cocaine.

The body shows withdrawal symptoms, like cocaine.

Also, the body shows a "high" in the brain after consuming food, like cocaine.

Eating when you're emotional creates genuine, physiological alleviation like taking a Valium.

These are all realities.

So why are individuals as yet suggesting to utilize resolve and discipline to battle cravings and beat the addiction to food?

If we realize that we wouldn't ever give a drug someone who is addicted the advice to "battle the craving" – why might we continue to give individuals who are dependent on food a similar advice?

It's basic: the general population who recommend that you utilize discipline clearly have never experienced this, and they don't genuinely understand the underlying science. It's shabby self help with no tried formula.

Chapter 22
Mind Tricks

Your whole approach has to be different from simply "fighting it."

Drug addicts need to discover that hanging out with their old companions doesn't work any longer. They have to change who they associate with – they do this because they realize that once they see companions doing drugs or smoking cigarettes, odds are they're going to need to, too.

You're fighting a genuine addiction. You must choose the option to think "keen" about how to beat it.

What I offer here are approaches to oversee – not some marvel cures.

For some individuals genuinely dependent on food, there is no such thing as moderation.

Also, for the most part, these fall into three general categories: behavioral shifts like changing your propensities and routines.

Psychological shifts, which involve your thinking about food.

And afterward nutritional shifts, which involve changing what kinds of foods you eat, and when.

These all genuinely rotate around training your mind in different approaches to be moreaware. Without mindfulness, it's tough to change.

So here are the 5 Jedi mind traps that really work.

Mental Hack #1: Figure Out Your Eating Type... And Then Dominate It

Although the categories aren't new, he put some cunning names that help you remember which kind of eater you are.

He separates individuals into 5 common groups:

A. The supper stuffer. Dinner stuffers eat basically during mealtimes, but they stuff themselves and eat to overabundance. They often eat so rapidly that they're uncomfortably full after. These are the kids we often say have "great cravings." They often backpedal for seconds.

B. Snack slow eater. Snack slow eaters go after food at whatever point it's accessible. Convenience is typically the main reason – in other words, food is accessible and they just constantly go after it as long as it's there. Snacking is sometimes an anxious propensity or something they do when exhausted. Sometimes they snack as a reason to get up and stroll around, or they simply feel "exhausted" when watching television or reading.

C. The gathering binger. Party bingers are typically professionals or individuals in corporate environments. Food is either a background for business or fun, and it's easy to forget about how much they eat or drink. Lots of social occasions and business meetings implies lots of food and eating out.

D. The restaurant indulger. Restaurant indulgers are individuals who regularly eat out a lot at restaurants. Sometimes these are recently youthful college kids, other circumstances they're youthful professionals who work a lot and don't have any desire to/don't have room schedule–wise to cook. In this way, they eat out 3x a day.

E. Desktop/dashboard diner. Desktop diners speed eat while multitasking on the PC or driving. They more often than not do it to save time, but also do it just to dodge the hassle of getting a genuine lunch. They're not occupied, they're quite recently unmotivated. When you ask them why they don't simply cook their own food or go get a genuine feast, they say "Eh… ."

So now you know your eating sort. You know your own kryptonite. You know for example you're a desktop diner. You know you are exceptionally unlikely to really eat a full supper while at work – and that you wind up eating a couple candy bans throughout the day from the vending machine, leaving you starving for dinner (despite the fact that you ate 1,000+ calories).

You know you are prone to not being set up for lunch. What's more, you realize that you for the most part feel too "sluggish" to go out for a dinner and wind up feasting on the vending machine. So what can you do?

You can consciously get ready lunch beforehand and bring it.

You can set a personal "administer" for yourself – make yourself go out to lunch with individuals at least twice every week.

Alternately you can set a run where you don't give yourself a chance to eat at your work area – to guarantee that you formally have some kind of lunch.

Suppose you're a nibbler.

You know you constantly go after food throughout the day and once in a while eat a full feast. You also realize that if there's a candy dish, you're most likely going to constantly have your hand it in throughout the day.

With that new mindfulness, you can do a couple things:

Set an alarm on your iPhone to remind yourself at regular intervals to eat a dinner.

Never, ever carry snacks with you – forcing yourself to eat dinners routinely.

Keep away from situations where you have the chance to constantly have your hands in the treat shake.

Along these lines, here's mental hack #1: Learn your eating sort (AKA your kryptonite) and after that be set up for those situations by having escape plans and strategically building your day around them.

Mental Hack #2: Emotional Learning

For some (most?) of us, emotional eating has become a propensity for comfort – in other words, it's a behavior induced by certain signs like situations, feelings, individuals, advertisements, and so on.

In studies, creatures and individuals that were more focused on wound up eating progressively and getting fatter.

In the vast dominant part of individuals, uncontrolled eating occurs in two (emotion–related) situations:

>•Boredom ("I'm quite recently sitting watching TV and eating")

>•Stress occasions ("I feel awful, so I eat")

So here's how you utilize emotional learning to adopt the keen strategy to beating food addiction, which ultimately rotates around your propensities.

I've beforehand discussed this a considerable amount in a post called 'Why all diets fizzle and why you don't require a diet to shed pounds, but here's a recap for emotional eaters.

Via Charles Duhigg's book The Power of Habit

#1 Figure Out Your Cues

The greater part of us emotionally eat because of prompts outside or inside of us.

For example: we're at an organization party. Food is there, so we eat it (accessibility – outside prompt).

Another example: It's 2:30 at work, and you're on the home extend. You begin getting low vitality, and you're looking for something to do – so you go upstairs to the bistro and get a treat (low vitality – internal prompt).

So the secret for a large portion of us is to A. take in our prompts, and afterward B. maintain a strategic distance from them.

A system I commonly recommend for figuring out your prompts is what I call the Awesomesauce Index Card Method.

•But to keep it basic, invest energy for 1–2 weeks recording a couple of things:

•What time do I pine for food?

•What states of mind make me need food? (Normally weariness and stress)

•In what situations do I as a rule over eat?

•With what individuals do I as a rule eat the wrong foods?

•What places more often than not wind up causing cravings?

#2 Swap The Routine

Another incredibly common origin of negative behavior patterns is weariness.

I once was working with a housewife who had sugar cravings, and after doing the index card practice for 1–2 weeks (see above), she understood that every last bit of her sugar consumption happened when was "exhausted" or wanting something to do.

While watching TV mindlessly, surfing the internet, or simply hanging out around the house, she simply needed something to do – which wound up turning into a massive sugar consumption propensity.

Fortunately for her, once she made sense of the signal, she changed the routine.

In this way, suppose you realize that you eat food when you're exhausted. You can do #1 (abstain from being exhausted), or when you're exhausted (and acknowledge it), begin doing something that gives you something to do.

For example: If, at work, 2:30 hits and you're getting somewhat exhausted and tired, and you know you for the most part go up to the bistro for a snack, find something to do that stimulates you. Maybe that implies stopping over at a companion's work area to chat for a while, or maybe that implies just strategically placing your lunch soften later up the day, or maybe that implies saving your most interesting projects for around that opportunity to keep your brain focused.

Strategy #2 all rotates around three things: the emotion you're feeling, why you're feeling it, and finding things that really address the underlying cause (e.g. weariness).

Mental Hack #3: Cognitive Control

Psychological control spins all around how you see food, and I separate it into two general categories:

1.Mental chatter

2.Personal standards

There's often a lot of self–talk going on when we attempt to battle foods (or battle anything, truly). Also, what for the most part winds up happening is that the additional time we attempt to talk ourselves out of something, the stronger it becomes and the more it takes our attention.

Ever had a go at jumping off a high rock? The longer you hold up and talk yourself up, the less possibility you will really hop.

One of the easiest things you can do with respect to your mind is change the mental chatter.

Rather than looking at treats and frozen yogurt and saying to yourself, "Goodness man those look great," disclose to yourself reality, "I know I can't simply have one nibble... I'm going to eat 20," and even remind yourself of your objectives, "tomorrow I'm going to feel like poop and totally lament this."

Jon Grant, at the college of Minnesota, asks patients with a history of shoplifting to work out a shopping list before they go to the supermarket and simply put two things on the rundown: handcuffs, to remind them of their past history, and a bologna sandwich, to remind them of what they were eating in prison.

Basically this fair refreshes their memory and reminds them of the consequences of their behavior, and like saying "I'll feel unpleasant after eating treats," it instills a feeling of blame beforehand. (Hat tip to The End of Overreating for this account).

Food Rules

Setting rules for your food is another approach to beat using self discipline.

For example, you can make rules like "I don't eat french fries," or "I don't snack."

Governs really aren't using self control – and they can rapidly become propensities which bypass determination altogether.

It's best just to pick 2 or 3 standards to adhere to, that you can apply in an assortment of situations. Better yet, look at hack #1, find your eating sort, and set guidelines based on what kind of eater you are.

My own most loved personal standards? I don't eat french fries or any seared foods and don't snack.

These rapidly become a piece of your character, and when you say "I don't eat french fries" it closes the conversation and doesn't require any fighting whatsoever.

Mental Hack #4: Leveraging Social

Your social networks can fuel your food addiction and contribute to being overweight.

A review done in the New England Journal of Medicine found that social networks can advance obesity – individuals with companions, siblings and spouses who are obese are considerably more likely to be obese themselves.

Presently, although this wasn't in reference to online social networks (where individuals may not see each other as a general rule), there is proof that shows that you're ordinarily more prone to have an indistinguishable interests from your companions.

This is recently the long method for saying that individuals have a tremendous influence over your prosperity or disappointment, and you're likely to wind up like the general population around you in more than one way.

You can use the internet social spheres to support you too. There are a couple innovative locales to help you integrate a constructive social environment with your own personal objectives.

Fitocracy

Fitocracy more or less: It's health and wellness, gamified. You win points for doing "journeys" (otherwise known as certain workouts/destinations/objectives), and after that you can level up and achieve new levels.

It integrates with a social bolster like facebook, and gives others a chance to motivate and bail each other out.

Stickk

Stickk more or less: Stickk is another approach to socially integrate betting with attaining your own objectives.

It's based all in all "carrot and stick" hypothesis of motivation – that to motivate individuals, you can offer them incentives ($$$), or rebuff them.

In Stickk, you set an objective, and after that pick your stakes: if you neglect to achieve your objective, your money will automatically be sent to either a companion, a philanthropy, or better yet – an anti-philanthropy, otherwise known as a philanthropy you hate.

The key is to pick a philanthropy you hate so much that you'd rather kick the bucket than see your money go there

It works!

Dietbet

Dietbet more or less: Dietbet is an approach to socially challenge your companions to a health challenge. It's basically like where all of you toss money in the pot, and the general population who get nearest to their objectives assert the cash. Truly sweet right?

Social betting gone advanced.

Beyond the online tools and assets to help you conquer emotional eating and food addiction, the point of mental hack #4 is to use individuals to use your prosperity.

If you need to gain control over your eating, figure out how to use individuals in couple ways:

> •Build a support group or hang out in online forums where individuals have a similar experience and objectives

> •Embark on a test with a companion (or your whole family)

> •State an objective... openly, and after that have loved ones expect you to remember (like the online projects I talked about)

Individuals, sometimes more than anything, influence your prosperity or disappointment.

Mental Hack #5: Become Your Own Coach

Anyone with a chronic health problem has immediately discovered that they have to become their own expert.

Beyond simply learning everything regarding the matter, you have to understand your own vulnerabilities, and begin experimenting.

It's practically difficult to truly concoct a perfect diet for each person, or a perfect framework for each person – which is the reason experimentation is so critical.

For example, if you realize that certain foods make you over eat each time – you know you have a personal kryptonite and you ought to avoid them.

So how specifically do you experiment and become your own expert?

Utilize something that I call "definitive documents."

I've unfortunately had a number of different health problems in my life that were chronic and extremely difficult to solve by western doctors. As a rule there were many pieces to the astound, and I was left experimenting on my own.For a number of you this will be a similar case. Over the years, I wound up creating these word documents called "definitive documents" where I could document each bit of the bewilder I was trying to solve:

What do you write in them? Everything you know.

For emotional eaters and individuals that are dependent on food, monitor the following things:

>•Events that trigger scenes; would you say you were out with family? Is it safe to say that you were at a business lunch? Is it safe to say that you were eating lunch alone? Did you not have time for lunch?

>•What kinds of foods are your kryptonite that you wind up craving

more than others? What foods do you over-eat, each time you eat them?

•Experiments you have attempted; does eating oatmeal for breakfast leave you full, or do eggs? What time do you generally get sugar cravings? What has worked to beat your sugar cravings?

We as a whole need to become our own expert, especially if we have a long-standing chronic problem – often there are numerous, many interconnected pieces that one person cannot give you.

Thought of a hypothesis or hypothesis, test it, and record the outcomes in your definitive document. It becomes your own little doctor's notebook.

20844086R00087

Printed in Great Britain
by Amazon